CELEBRATING YOUR VIBRANT FUTURE

Intermittent Fasting for Women 44 to Forever

LAURIE LEWIS
WITH KIM SMITH

An Unbelievable Freedom Book

Copyright © 2020 Laurie Lewis and Kim Smith
All rights reserved.
Cover Artwork: Ameya Okamoto.
Author Photograph: Sarah Waters.
Designed and formatted by Eled Cernik.
ISBN-13: 979-8-6191180-5-6

For Mom,

*Thank you for my life,
your transcendent love,
and the miraculous words,*

"How may I support you?"

"...let your light so shine..."

MATTHEW 5:16

Table of Contents

Welcome from Kim 7

HELLO! 9

FOUNDATION

44 – 54 11
Creating Your Second Half 13
Why Daily Fasting? 20
How Does It Work? 22
Myths & Misconceptions 25
Fasting: The Clean Fast 27
Fasting: Clean Fast Chart 28
Fasting: Schedules 29
Eating: The Right Foods 32
Concerns & What to Expect 34
Adjustment Phase Bingo 36
Measuring Progress 37
Weighing 39
Wins 43

FAST FORWARD

How to Use the Daily Log 45

Week One: Let's Do This 46

Week Two: The Push 52

Week Three: The Bold Stretch 58

Week Four: Noticing-Noticing-Noticing 64

Week Five: My Sweet Spot 70

Week Six: Hitting My Stride 76

Week Seven: Taking Stock 82

Week Eight: A New Stretch 88

Week Nine: Great Way to Live 94

Week Ten: Considering My Future 100

Week Eleven: No Turning Back 106

Week Twelve: Next Level 112

FAST FOREVER

Troubleshooting 119

Discouragement 122

Maintenance 122

Your Vibrant Future 123

Take it From Here: Resources 125

Love Letters *to* You 127

Cheers *from* Laurie 133

Welcome from Kim

Greetings!

And just like that, we are publishing the 13th Unbelievable Freedom Habit Guide! Like several before it, it deals with the powerful health practice called intermittent fasting. The book is *Celebrating Your Vibrant Future: Intermittent Fasting for Women 44 to Forever* and its author, Laurie Lewis, is one of my original "fasting friends" met in 2017 in the Delay, Don't Deny Facebook community. Since that time, I've become an author and publisher, and Laurie has become an inspirational, impactful IF coach.

Since I know thousands of intermittent fasters, including multiple IF coaches, why did I choose Laurie to bring her writing to the series? Plainly stated, Laurie has more passion for the art & science of fasting than anyone I know. As we've worked side by side to encourage members in the Delay, Don't Deny community online, I've been awed by Laurie's dedication and drive to support others. She willingly shares both her personal journey with health transformation and her ever-expanding knowledge of IF research.

Laurie is the first person I approached to become an Unbelievable Freedom collaborator, and I'm so pleased the day is finally here. I'm applauding her contribution and you'll soon be celebrating your vibrant future!

Enjoy Your Life,
Kim

KIM SMITH is a believer in the inspirational power of story and the transformational power of habits. She's the Creative Director of Unbelievable Freedom, LLC, and the curator of the Unbelievable Freedom Habit Guide Series. She is also proud to be the Poster Girl for Contentment.

Hello!

This book is a hug.

Wherever you are on the trajectory of "44 to forever," dear reader, I suspect that some point along the way you questioned, Is it *really* downhill from here? Will I just succumb to feeling sicker, heavier, and foggier? Do I have to take more and more medications to survive? Even with life's immeasurable joys, will my unique self disappear into a future of discomfort and struggle?

Menopause crushed me.

Perhaps, the mental and physical surprises starting in your late 40's were startling for you? They were for me. If you aren't there yet, you are possibly wondering, "What the heck is coming? Can I escape it?" Good questions! Nobody sent us to biology class for aging women, and we have been left to figure it out on our own. It does not help that the mention of "menopause" will silence and embarrass a room; notice how people *whisper* the word.

Or, if menopause is spoken of at all, it is treated as a joke; as if depression, raging heat, wobbly balance, debilitating confusion, serious forgetfulness, lack of sex-drive, and surges of sadness and anger are any laughing matter. I didn't find it funny. I found it embarrassing, horrifying, disorienting, and frightening. The only way I could describe it was that an alien had taken over my body and spirit. Ever the optimist, I struggled to maintain sporadic glimmers of hope; I worked to envision a magical return to myself.

I fantasized that this five-year perimenopausal hell would end when my monthly cycle finally ceased. *That* was indeed the joke. When my period bid adieu at age 49, I suddenly packed on 50+ pounds of stubborn, hormonal fat. Nothing worked to turn it around, and needless to say, I was determined. I used all my nutrition training + old weight-loss tricks from running to juice fasts, from low carb programs to eliminating foods that sparked a "hormonal response." Little did I know, *all* foods elicit hormonal responses and my old tricks were not going to work. I had a lot to learn! People in my life were baffled, "How could *you* gain so much weight? You're the healthiest person we know!" Those thoughts and messages compounded my fears that it truly must be *all downhill from here.*

Yet, it all turned out. After 4.5 years of trying to right the ship, I reached a point of utter hopelessness. Despondent is just about the right description, and at the onset of a long visit home to visit my mother, she lovingly encouraged that "we use this time to turn the weight around." (*eeeek!*) What followed was a tearful, explosive conversation, culminating in her offer to pray for an answer. I accepted the kindness, and ascended the stairs for yet another desperate googling session of "menopause women stubborn fat loss diet hormones help me." I will never know what happened, but my heart sings with gratitude that on *that* night, the words "Intermittent Fasting" popped up for the first time.

I was familiar with long, therapeutic fasting, having been fascinated by Upton Sinclair's 1911 book, "The Fasting Cure." But, I had no clue that a person could live a life of daily fasting. The first videos I watched were by the prolific and upbeat, Dy Ann Parham. She had just ramped up her thrice-weekly video series, and I was hooked. I dove down the rabbit hole watching Dr. Eric Berg and Dr. Jason Fung. As the sun peeked over the Colorado ridgelines, I could not wait to head downstairs to inform my mom that the answer had come. I knew 100% what I was going to do.

"I'm going to stop eating for a portion of every day. This practice will balance my hormones and give my body a much-needed opportunity to heal every day. I will eat lunch and dinner, and maybe pretty soon, I will only have dinner. If I start feeling sick or acting weird, I'll stop right away. What do you think?"

"I think it sounds like a great idea! How may I support you?"

Never missing a day of fasting, I shed the 50+ pounds in 15 months, fitting easily into all the clothing I wore so happily in 2012. Over 1,000 fasts and three years later, I have a thriving coaching and workshop business (Fast Forward Wellness) based on my personal success with and love of Intermittent Fasting. A highlight has been working alongside Gin Stephens, author of "Delay, Don't Deny: Living an Intermittent Fasting Lifestyle," joyfully coaching thousands upon thousands of new fasters to be successful with their fasting regimens.

I like stories and I like science, but what I *really* like is a linear progression from A to Z. Therefore, I have taken my personal fasting journey, piled up the countless books, podcasts, videos, articles, and scientific research I have dug into, and designed a three-month plan for every woman "44 to forever" who is ready to own her wellness.

Having a daily fasting regimen *is* the underlying foundation for health, freedom, aliveness, joy, discernment, awakening, pleasure, and peace-of-mind.

The practice is 100% experiential, meaning, it is impossible to fully describe the magic that takes place in one's body, mental state, and emotions when you pause from eating. That is precisely why I accepted Kim Smith's invitation to write for her Unbelievable Freedom workbook series. This compilation will take you from start to success, and you will chart, question, scribble, scream, ruminate, remember, draw, and track your path.

I have four key intentions for this workbook. You will:

- Discover fasting as an awakening which provides freedom and vitality
- Experience newfound honor, joy, wonder, and curiosity in this next phase of your life
- Feel enlivened, connected, beautiful, respected, and appreciated
- Be in action, consistent, and purposeful

You will learn to:

- Eat in a pattern of time
- Eat foods you love, and choose the foods that love you back
- Eat the right quantities of food to satiety
- Fully enjoy the pleasure and nourishment of food
- Relish in the healing and peace-of-mind that fasting provides
- Kick "diet mindset" to the curb
- Successfully fast every day – even with vacations, festivities, and life's stresses
- Reap the countless and unimaginable benefits available from fasting

Please know that you are not washed up, over, finished, invisible, deteriorating, or done. **You're ready!** Wherever you are in this journey of "44 to forever," we are taking the next steps together.

Cheers to your vibrant future!

Foundation

44 - 54

Welcome to this most extraordinary next phase of your life! Before we embark on the Intermittent Fasting instructions, let's get grounded in where you are, or where you may have been.

Why is 44 our starting point?

I awoke one night in the fall of 2007 and thought, "It's a thousand degrees in here. I need to buy a new air conditioner!" At 44, that was my first realization of perimenopause. A more mystical answer to "Why 44?" is that in March of 2017, a few months before learning about Intermittent Fasting, I saw 44 elephants in one day while scouring the landscape in South Africa. In many cultures, 44 is an auspicious number, considered the master healer, related to building something that will benefit future generations.

Which, most importantly, leads to you. Forty-four is for you who have not yet experienced any signs of "the change," but you know it is coming and you want to tackle aging head on. This is not meant to be alarming, but rather, awakening and empowering. I can point to countless women in my life who experienced debilitating health concerns right around age 47-48, so addressing your health at 44 is inspiring and wise.

Forty-four is also for those of you who may be well past 44, who are remembering your early 40's with fondness, or horror, or perhaps a smidge of regret. You may certainly skip ahead to the next section, but perhaps a stroll down memory lane – 44-54 – is in order. Whether you are peering ahead or reflecting, let's briefly look together at this mystery called menopause.

Can we agree that the majority of us were never educated about this phenomenon? While these pages do not displace more involved medical study, they are an overview of the symptoms.

The years before menopause are called perimenopause, which indicates a major shift in the hormones estrogen, progesterone, and testosterone. Women may experience:

- Fatigue
- Night sweats
- Hot flashes and sweating
- Irregular menstrual cycles
- Shorter cycles
- Longer than normal cycles
- Extreme bleeding
- Bloating not just pre-cycle
- Decreased libido
- Painful sex
- Dry hair and hair loss
- Brittle fingernails
- Increase in anxiety
- Surges in depression
- Irritability
- Incontinence
- Joint pain
- Frozen shoulder
- Sleeplessness

- Memory loss
- Loss of balance and dizzy spells
- Trouble concentrating
- New allergies or food sensitivities
- Irregular heartbeat
- Osteoporosis
- Onset of autoimmune diseases
- Stress-related adrenal fatigue
- Weight gain

This isn't for the faint of heart, and I don't need to remind you, it isn't a joke. This certainly may not be true for every woman, and we bow in amazement at women whose periods have suddenly stopped one day without a signal, and they carry on as if nothing happened. If that happens to be you, one of our 54+ readers, happy dance and high fives all around!

Go through the list thoughtfully and honestly my 44 – 54 gals. There is nothing "wrong" with you. Your body is embarking on its next magnificent phase, and anyone who can get through *this* is one tough mama!

Now is a good time to **begin marking up this book**. *Find your favorite sparkly pen or highlighter, and circle, underline, and jot down questions about some of the challenges you may be experiencing.*

Our bodies hold over 50 different hormones and they are each chemical messengers operating in a hierarchy with their unique connections and balance. They are the foundation for healthy mood, appetite, sex drive, clear thinking, focus, and over-all well-being. So the next time you have a critical thought about being "too hormonal," think again... you are magnificently hormonal!

I have *three important instructions*:

1. Once you have reviewed and marked up this list, **call a friend** and have an open conversation about menopause. Speaking about it, and helping one another, is an important step in understanding and accepting what is happening. Make a pact to *never whisper* "menopause" again.

2. **Make an appointment** with your health care practitioner, and before the visit, study up! Perhaps you are a lucky woman who has a physician who will listen, request the hormonal tests, and offer support. Sadly, most women 44-54 are dismissed as over-reacting. If you learn through your research that you suspect you should be having tests for Thyroid (TSH, free T3, free T4, reverse T3), Cortisol, Testosterone, Progesterone, Estrogen, etc., be armed with questions, knowledge, and be ready to make some powerful requests. Your doctor works for you.

3. **Start Intermittent Fasting today.** Good! That's why you have this book in your hands. If you're 44, this is an exciting time, and as a woman who Intermittent Fasts you just may be able to mitigate or avoid many of these challenges. Remember, the body is always working towards homeostasis, which means that even our beloved and temperamental hormones can eventually arrive in their perfectly-tuned balanced state.

You are the boss. Sending the power of 44 your way!

Creating Your Second Half

You are holding this workbook, so you are already a solid YES! As I envision your commitment to your vitality, I match it with my promise to guide and support. You inspire me, and together we are going to rock this 100%.

When it comes to using this workbook, I have four types of fasting friends who use this tool quite differently. They are The Rebel, The Writer, The Sponge, and The Talker.

Nina, the Rebel, uses this workbook *her* way, scribbling one word for each question. She is zipping forward, and bulleted responses suffice. The only reason she is writing anything at all is because there are some things she knows she does not want to forget.

Deborah, the introverted Writer, uses the workbook methodically as a private safe haven. She finds solace in meticulously downloading experiences and ideas. Every square inch is filled with reflections. Using the workbook is therapeutic.

Amanda, the "gotta learn everything" Sponge, views the workbook as a scaffolding. She then spans out to absorb all the videos, books, podcasts, studies, and articles she can find so she can build her practice. This workbook is the place to capture all she is learning.

Vanessa, the Talker, comes alive when she is sharing and listening with others. The workbook works for her if she can meet with a friend, share, write, inquire, inspire, uplift, and hold one another to account.

How will you use this workbook as a tool to best support you? You get to say.

This process is tailored to your life, your body, your desires... and I'm here... listening.

Perimenopause and menopause are a time of awakening. This new phase is a liberation, it is a threshold that opens wide a new view of our body, of our life, of our womanhood.

Look closely at how things currently are for you regarding your weight, wellness, vitality. **Take the time to reflect and document** what has happened, what things looks like for you now, what it feels like now, and how you want to feel.

If you have ever had a hunch that we have been sold a bill of goods about our age, our beauty, our visibility, our sexiness, our nutrition, our fitness, and our importance, please use these next few pages to examine, write, and draw what you are observing and experiencing.

The biggest thing I'm dealing with is:

The words to describe how I feel are:

I am most afraid of:

Draw what you feel like here, or cut out a photograph from a magazine that illustrates your current feelings about your body and yourself. Stick it here with glue or tape:

Let's look at commitment. You are here because you have valid reasons and you are motivated. Let's dig into some possible degrees and styles of motivation. Where might you find yourself?

Urgently: Your health is at risk and you have a serious diagnosis. It is required that you take action and not deviate.

Highly: You feel despondent, hopeless, at the end of your rope. You have tried everything and need to make immediate changes. You will do whatever it takes.

Seriously: You are exasperated and tired of feeling poorly, but do not have a "take no prisoners" attitude. You want to reap the results, yet desire little pressure or few life alterations. You will trust the process because you are confident that small steps aggregate into major shifts and healing.

Pleasantly: You are already feeling free, fit, and well, and you embrace daily fasting as a feasible way to live. You will apply the clean fasting techniques, and your approach is one of zero stress and minor tweaks.

It is likely that you see yourself in a few places. Please take the time to examine and write where you stand regarding motivation:

Dieting is brutal. My diet history included a horrifying summer of the 330 calorie-per-day Cambridge Diet, years off and on Slim Fast, juice fasts and the master cleanse, and a very random I ♥ NY Diet chosen purely because of my love of NYC. All I remember of that diet were lots of strawberries. Weird.

Write some of the diets and weight-loss schemes that you have endured here:

These next questions are tough to contemplate without assigning fault and blame. If you can — I know you can — please take stock of how you got here. What happened?

Without making yourself wrong, can you identify some aspects of your health or diet history that contributed to the current challenges? It could be as simple as, "Menopause hit, my hormones went haywire, and I didn't know what to do." Or, it could look like, "I have tried every diet on earth since I was 8 years old, and I can't take it any more, so I eat ALL the things and then beat myself up." Or, "I have a high-stress life, I am overwhelmed, it never ends, so I eat on the fly and make terrible choices."

Take the case it is not your "fault." Our hormones, primarily insulin, cortisol, leptin, and ghrelin are out of balance and calling the shots. In the climate of calorie-restriction, over-exercising, and eating at all hours, we cannot win. So, if we take "fault" out of the equation, *what happened* for you? How did we get here?

What will make this journey successful for me?

Where do I anticipate snags and snarls?

What might I do or say to myself when I want to quit?

Where might I let myself down or let myself off the hook?

What am I willing to do differently now?

What do I most wish for myself, my body, my life right now?

I'm done with beating and wrestling my body into submission. If I stopped hating it, what *could* I think about it?

If my 20's and 30's were about being perfect and getting it "right," what could my 40's and 50's be used for?

What could 60, 70, 80, 90, and 100+ be for? Write some new "themes" for each decade:

Even when I am struggling, who in my world needs me now? List all of the areas in your life where you are needed and valuable.

If you consider a new venture or idea as a "spark," **who in your life are your "Spark Tenders"?** Who will encourage you and cheer you on? Be judicious about who you share with, because some people are well-meaning soul crushers. In the beginning, you only want people who will tend to this spark and help you keep it aflame.

Who is the person who believes in you long before you believe in yourself?

Write a few names, or just one, here. And, if that one person is me, it will be our secret. Feel free to email me and let me know. I am your Spark Tender.

You have allowed yourself to begin dreaming, and you're clear that this is a starting point. You are turning a corner. Well done. Now, let's immerse ourselves in what brought you here, the allure and promise of Intermittent Fasting.

Why Daily Fasting?

I suspect that the reason you are here with me, digging into this workbook, is because somebody told you about the benefits of Intermittent Fasting. Maybe you observed that person from afar, and you want what they are experiencing. Or, perhaps you saw a news report, article, video, or scientific journal. I have a hunch that you already have a bit of knowledge. Hooray for your inspired curiosity!

Intermittent Fasting is akin to how we evolved and survived as humans. Quite simply, it is only in recent times that human beings have had 24/7 access to fully stocked fridges. We blindly consider food availability and eating patterns "normal," yet our alarming obesity rates coupled with the commonplace nature of lifestyle diseases (cardiovascular disease, type 2 diabetes, etc.) are killing us. Literally.

We are trying very hard and have been stressed and strained. We have been in a hamster wheel attempting to lose weight (whether it's 10 pounds or 200) and we are ravenously fixated on food, eating too much, measuring, berating ourselves, sneaking, deprived, dissatisfied, resentful, and unsuccessful. This is no way to live, and it is not how human beings are designed.

This is far from normal, acceptable, or sustainable. Nobody wants to live with this level of discomfort and illness, yet we have not yet been aware enough to announce: We need a period of metabolic and digestive rest. We need to stop eating all the time. We need to fast for healing every day.

Remind me again, what is your number one reason for starting Intermittent Fasting? Please, **write that reason here:**

Now, please, scour the following lists, **circle what resonates**, and **add bullet points** of your own.

The (serious) benefits of daily fasting – I.F. isn't messing around:

- Prevent and reverse diseases, such as cancer, autoimmune diseases, cardiovascular disease, alzheimer's, type 2 diabetes, metabolic syndrome, asthma, multiple sclerosis, arthritis
- Resist cellular damage
- Improve memory and cognitive function
- Slow the progression of neurological degradation
- Heal tissue damage
- Increase effectiveness of chemotherapy and other healing modalities
- Restore and balance the gut microbiome
- Gain in physical strength and performance
- Utilize body fat for energy
- Restore the body's natural and healthy set weight point
- Lengthen lifespan

Life gets easier – these improvements would change so much for us:

- Normalize blood pressure
- Normalize blood sugar
- Achieve healthy cholesterol numbers
- Heal digestion and gut issues
- Eliminate aching joints
- Smooth out wrinkles, bumps, scars

- Enjoy foods without acid reflux
- Respond to stress without using food to cope
- Climb, step, and run with ease
- Enjoy an even-keel energy throughout the day
- Sleep more soundly
- Walk easily without the pain of plantar fasciitis
- Speed up your metabolic rate
- Settle into a "normal" BMI and body fat percentage
- Reverse symptoms of menopause

The ordinary and thrilling – seems too good to be true:

- Have an even, peaceful temperament
- Enjoy foods without calculating calories, points, and macronutrients. Just eat!
- Sit for hours during a conference without your ankles swelling
- Slip on your wedding rings again
- Recognize yourself in the mirror
- Have fun shopping for new clothes
- Put your shoes on without sitting down
- Have people tell you your skin is glowing
- Feel comfortable in front of a camera
- Clip your toenails without holding your breath
- Zip up those tall boots
- Wear that cute skirt from 1983 that is back in style
- Fly without the extender seatbelt
- Have those skin tags and eye floaters disappear
- Don't worry about when you're eating next
- Clean up fewer dishes
- Easily get up off the floor with the dog or grandkids
- Save money
- No more thinking "food is bad," so, "I am bad," and "I have to be good"

Please write a bit more about what you now see is possible for you. Your goals could fall into three categories:

1. What matters most to me is:

2. It would be amazing if:

3. I can barely imagine, but it would be cool if:

How Does It Work?

Let's keep this simple, and save the long descriptions for the New England Journal of Medicine. There are countless articles, videos, and books where you can add to your knowledge, but trust me, the following information will sufficiently arm you in case your critical co-worker warns that you are on a dangerous, metabolism-crushing, starvation diet.

There are seven main parts to remember.

Insulin

Insulin is a hormone made by the pancreas. Its function is to regulate blood sugar and then convert any unused glucose into glycogen and fat.

An over-abundance of circulating insulin (caused by frequent eating) leads to an issue called Insulin Resistance. This means that the cells are requesting insulin to manage blood sugar, but access is locked, thus leaving the body with an excess of insulin while the cells are screaming for more. Chaotic and unworkable!

The presence of insulin hinders the body's ability to access stored fat. When we are eating and drinking constantly, the body cannot tap into its fat stores. Remember, the primary reason we have fat in the first place is so we have readily available fuel in case of famine.

All foods, especially sweet tastes, elicit an insulin response. During our fasting hours, our aim is to keep insulin low, become insulin sensitive, and access our stored body fat for energy.

Energy/Fuel

Your body uses one fuel source at a time. It is not like a hybrid car, skating between fuel sources. It uses glucose (from what you just ate), glycogen (stored glucose), and then stored body fat. In that order. 1 – 2 – 3...

It can take several weeks to chip away at the stored glycogen in your liver. Even more is packed away in your muscles, and you will get to that deeper level in a few months. But for now, fast long and clean every day with the goal of reducing the glycogen in the liver, and then accessing your stored fat.

For now, remember glucose, glycogen, fat. 1 – 2 – 3...

Oh, and take note, the liver doesn't fill completely back up with glycogen every time you eat. Once you've depleted the glycogen stores, and you fast long and clean every day, your body will easily slip into fat burning. That, ladies, is being metabolically flexible!

Fat and Ketosis

Hooray! Approximately twelve hours after eating, the body has used up the glucose and shifts to utilizing glycogen. Then, a few hours after that (give or take) any remaining stores of glycogen are depleted, and you can finally switch into breezing along on your stored fat.

Except. Wait! Not so quick. It does *not* want to. The body, with the growling hormone ghrelin leading the charge, would prefer that you feed it. It *d e m a n d s* easy glucose.

However, if you stick to your guns, get through the feelings of hunger and mental anguish, your body will get the message and make that shift into using your body fat for energy.

Note* In case you panicked about my use of the phrase, "mental anguish," fear not! The deafening racket diminishes within the first weeks of practicing your fasting regimen. Phew. None of us need all that clatter. Bring on the peace-of-mind that comes with being in a fat-burning state!

Well done, you are now metabolically flexible. When those fats release from your fat cells, wind their way through your blood to your liver, they emerge in the form of ketone bodies. Those ketones are a mighty efficient fuel source, and "being in ketosis" is an extraordinary brain boost. This is the reason many daily fasters feel awake, sharp, and focused around eighteen hours fasted. The brain is fueling on ketones... a byproduct of your stored body fat.

If you notice a sweet, metallic, odd acetone taste in your mouth, or funny-smelling urine, this is an indication that the body is releasing ketones. It is fabulous news! Very shortly, excess ketone levels will drop as the body increases its ability to efficiently utilize ketones as fuel.

Autophagy

When in a fasted state, the body ramps up a cellular clean up process called autophagy. Damaged cell components are disassembled and the junky old proteins are recycled to build new materials. The freshly spruced-up cells are *so* perfect, in fact, that under a microscope, scientists cannot discern between the efficiently-repaired cells and brand new cells.

It is as if your rusty, broken down car were professionally detailed immaculately such that you could not tell the difference between your old car and a sparkling new car on the sales lot. That is really cleaned up!

What this means for you? Restored tendons, stronger bones, smoother skin, to name a few. One easy way to know that autophagy is at work is to notice scars, bumps, skin tags, and moles disappearing. If all that is occurring on your surface, imagine what is transforming deep down.

Pro Tip: Autophagy also "eats up" the excess skin as you lose fat. So, there's that to look forward to!

Human Growth Hormone (HGH)

This key hormone stimulates cell reproduction and generation, and also regulates body composition, mental function, sugar and fat metabolism, as well as muscle and bone growth.

Spikes in insulin (eating) disrupt our natural HGH production. However, when we are in the fasted state, HGH skyrockets 1000+% for women, resulting in stronger bones and toned muscles. This is occurs without hitting the gym. Miraculous, right?

Metabolism

No discussion about how Intermittent Fasting works would be complete without a chat about metabolic rate. Simply said, when the body perceives sufficient fuel (food, glucose, glycogen, body fat) the metabolic rate increases. When it senses a fuel deficit, the metabolism lowers. The body wants to do its job of keeping you alive, so it always raises or lowers the metabolic rate to match its perception of the availability of fuel. Basically, it is always asking, is there a famine, or isn't there?

For the dieter who is on a calorie-restriction plan, their circulating insulin is kept constantly high, so they rarely tap into their fat stores. Sadly, they never fully enjoy their tiny-frequent diet meals, they aren't eating to fullness, they aren't burning their stored fat, their body perceives a low level of food, and the body responds by lowering the metabolism.

But, for fasters who fast clean every day, our bodies have low circulating insulin; we tap into our fat for fuel, *and* we are eating abundant, satisfying foods. This combination of utilizing body fat for fuel, coupled with eating very well to satiety, increases the metabolic rate.

Appetite Correction

Fasting provides the opportunity to restore the brain-body connection. Deep in our brains we have an appetite control center, the appestat. Due to our constant consumption of meals, snacks, and snack-drinks, the hunger hormones and appestat are malfunctioning. This corrects when we pause from eating. In a few weeks you will begin to see evidence of, as Dr. Bert Herring calls it, "Appetite Correction" at play.

Some signs are: you won't be interested in foods you have been drawn to in the past, ultra-processed foods may taste odd, you might have strong thoughts of foods you have never liked (broccoli! brussels sprouts! squash!), you will not be able to eat your entire meal, *or*, on some days, your body will inform you it wants ALL the food! The appestat informs you of what to eat and how much to eat, and it varies from day to day.

This is one of the reasons that calorie counting is futile. After fasting clean for a few weeks, you will experience first-hand that the quantity of food your body requests is different every day. You will be losing fat without willpower or calorie counting. Your body, its appestat and hunger hormones, are in the driver's seat. And, all this is possible due to fasting.

Quick Review:

1. Fast Clean
2. Keep insulin low
3. Use up glucose, glycogen, and access stored body fat
4. Transform body fat into ketones to fuel the brain
5. Dramatically increase autophagy
6. Skyrocket the production of human growth hormone
7. Elevate metabolism
8. Repair the appetite center in the brain
9. BAM! You know what is happening.

Myths & Misconceptions

Of course, we can foresee moments when the naysayers and ne'er-do-wells – who have skimmed nothing but headlines – will spout their sensationalism and cause you to doubt what you know. It is ok. I predicted those types too. I was so uncertain in my first months that I told nobody other than my mother. I did not have the bandwidth to adequately describe or defend, even when I was confident that I was feeling exceptionally well and my fasting regimen was working.

When you are ready to let some people know that you now eat in a pattern, on a schedule, that you are an Intermittent Faster, you may want to embolden yourself with a few more answers.

"You are starving yourself."

The definition of starvation is to "suffer or die from lack of food." Fasting every day matches the design of humans, and I have plenty of food to eat when it is time to eat. Also, I can choose to break my fast any time I please. I move my eating window around to match my life. Also, have you *seen* me eat? Starvation? Hardly!

"Fasting will ruin your metabolism."

My body is tapping into my own fat stores for fuel, plus I am eating delicious, abundant meals. When the body knows there is an abundance of fuel, the metabolism goes up."

"Your body will target muscle for fuel."

As Dr. Jason Fung says, "the body is not that stupid." Its primary energy sources are glycogen and fat. I am nowhere near running out of fat! Since my body is now a fat burning machine, *and* I'm building muscle with the increase in HGH, I have no worries that my body is working exactly as designed. Muscle Up! Fat Down!

"The only way you can know how much to eat is by counting calories or points."

I take the case that my brain is as savvy as a giraffe's or a lion's. Wild animals are perfectly fit and lean, and they don't count calories. Fasting is healing the appetite sensors in my brain are informing me exactly how much food the body needs every day. Some days I eat more food, other days I eat less food. Exactly as designed!

Look at all the misery and crazy-making that calorie and points counting has caused. Not to mention, the abysmal success-rate. We are more sick and obese than we have ever been. I am learning to listen and trust my body.

"I'm not sure this will be a good example for my children."

Children understand that they are growing and should eat when they are hungry. As adults, we are no longer growing. We practice eating in an "eating window" and it is fun for them to help remind us when our window is open and when it is closed.

I figure the best example is to teach them to eat when they are hungry and do not force food upon anyone. Have food available for them when they get hungry. Remember our parents used to say, "No snacking! You will ruin your dinner"? That was a really good rule. Eat meals with no grazing or late-night snacking. When dinner is over, it is over.

It is helpful for us to model empowering thoughts and words regarding food. Food isn't bad, we are not bad, nor are we good for eating certain foods. We don't need to hide food or demonize it. Food is food. Some foods make us feel well and perform well. Other foods do not. We will be mindful of choosing foods that make us feel great! And, we always make sure we fully enjoy what we are eating. Mangia!

"This plan is simply calorie-restriction. You're eating less, so of course you will lose weight."

Some days I eat less food and some days more. In research studies, when two groups of subjects are given the same amount of food — some eat it spread out over the day, and the other group eats it in a shorter window — the time-restricted subjects lose more weight *and* are happier with the plan.

Spreading small amounts of food out throughout the day never leaves us satisfied, and we feel hungrier and unable to tap into our fat stores. Intermittent fasting isn't about calories. Eating food in an eating window allows us to tap into our fat stores *and* enjoy our delicious food.

Also, I am not only interested in losing weight, I am inspired by *all* of the healing that intermittent fasting provides.

"I heard that fasting messes with a woman's hormones."

Billions of women have fasted every day throughout human history. Our survival has depended on it. Given the main hormone that fasting effects is insulin, and it is detrimental to our health to have high levels of circulating insulin, women should implement a fasting regimen to keep insulin low and ward off metabolic syndrome.

Fasting actually restores the health of our endocrine system. Personally, fasting balanced my estrogen, progesterone, and testosterone. Fasting lowered my circulating insulin and cortisol, and enabled my hunger hormones ghrelin and leptin to function correctly. Fasting provides healing repair and creates balance.

"I read that people with (fill in the blank) should not fast."

There is a short list of people for whom a strict fasting plan is not recommended: children, pregnant women, breast-feeding women, those with a history of disordered eating, and people with type one diabetes.

There are impressive accounts where patients with T1 have worked closely with their physicians to regulate their insulin, and they have successfully crafted a fasting schedule. This requires careful planning and close monitoring. Other than that, for those with adrenal fatigue, thyroid challenges, lyme disease, and so forth, fasting actually fills our tanks. Make sure the fasting schedule is not stress inducing, that it is peaceful, and you will see how fasting is restorative and regenerative.

"You will never be able to enjoy parties, vacations, brunches."

Sure, I will! I can plan to extend my eating window, or I can move it to the morning, midday, or late night. I travel fasted – water only — arriving at my destination refreshed with no jet lag. I enjoy hikes, cruises, beach excursions, wedding weekends, music festivals, road trips, amusement parks, conferences, tailgating, religious holidays, baby showers, and birthday parties. Cheers!

The best defense is your own experience. In very short order, the number one answer you will provide is, *"Thank you for your concern, but, I have never felt better and I am living a great life."*

Steel your resolve. Don't apologize or shrink. You know what you are doing. Enjoy!

Fasting: The Clean Fast

For an intermittent faster, there are two parts to every day, the fasting hours and the eating window.

You would think this would be starkly obvious. Fasting is fasting, and consuming anything – food or food-like — is not fasting. But, it is not that obvious. Suffice to say, human beings looooove to bend rules, and when it comes to fun flavors, we seem to wail for them aaaallllll the time.

Gin Stephens saved the day by coining the term and defining The Clean Fast. Her 2016 bestseller, "Delay, Don't Deny: Living an Intermittent Fasting Lifestyle" has supported hundreds of thousands of people in the "Delay Don't Deny" method of clean fasting. We know that clean fasting works.

Put down your candy-coffee and entertaining snack-drinks. Fast clean, and you will be keeping insulin low and accessing your stored body fat.

When you sneak in added flavors (gum, lemon, ginger, apple cider vinegar, cream, coconut oil, fruity waters, flavored teas, vanilla coffee, calorie-free sodas, pre-workouts, etc.) you will be sending "incoming food" signals to the brain. Insulin is mobilized, hunger hormones are alerted, and the digestive process is revved up.

RED ALERT! You do not want that.

You want to fast clean for two main reasons:

1. Access your stored body fat.
2. Clean fasting is much easier. Easier is better.

I have met hundreds of people who started their fasting regimen with added flavors, only to report easier fasting hours and quicker results once they started fasting clean. (HA! I am one of those people!)

The morning I informed my mother "I'm now an Intermittent Faster," I scooted straight over to the health food store and loaded up on fancy detox teas. I purchased five different tea concoctions, just to keep it interesting. (*Hello, Laurie!* The fasting hours are not supposed to be "interesting." Save the nourishing fun for the eating window.) It took me weeks to figure out that those teas were making me ravenously cranky and spiking my insulin. I cut them out, drank water and black coffee only, and the fasting hours became easy breezy.

- Plain, unflavored **water** of any temperature or sparkliness
- Plain, unflavored "black" **coffee** with nothing added
- Plain, unflavored "black" or "green" **tea** with nothing added
- Plain, unflavored **minerals**/electrolytes (magnesium, sodium, etc.)
- **Medications** as prescribed

Fasting clean is a badge of honor. And, it works. Don't mess around with it. Stick to the Yes column of the Clean Fast Chart. Period.

Gin Stephens' CLEAN FAST Chart

Yes!

- Water *(Unflavored)*
- Black coffee *(Unflavored)*
- Black or green tea, actual "tea leaves" only *(Unflavored)*
- Mineral water, club soda, sparkling or seltzer water *(Unflavored)*
- Minerals/electrolytes such as magnesium or salt *(Unflavored)*
- Medications *(As prescribed by your healthcare provider)*

Maybe...

We call this the "grey area." These items may cause an insulin response for some people

- Herbal tea *(Bitter flavor only)*
- Peppermint essential oil *(One drop for breath freshening only, NOT for water-enhancing)*
- Nitro Cold Brew Coffee *(Even if it's black)*
- Some vitamins and supplements *(There is no easy answer for all vitamins and supplements. Plain minerals are in the "Yes" column, and if they are food-like or listed in the "No" column, move them to your eating window.)*

No!

- Food
- Flavored water
- Flavored coffee
- Fruity, sweet, or matcha teas
- Diet sodas *(Even with 0 calories)*
- Natural or artificial flavors
- Food-like flavors of any type *(Fruit-juices, fruit flavors, etc.)*
- Apple cider vinegar
- Bone broth, broth, bouillon
- Added fats *(Including MCT oil, coconut oil, butter, etc.)*
- Cream, creamers, milk *(Any amount or variety)*
- Supplements *(Such as BCAA's, collagen, pre-workouts, exogenous ketones, etc.)*

Fasting: Schedules

The second question I am always asked after, "How do I not die of starvation?" is, "What is the best fasting schedule?"

Answer: I have no idea what is best for you.

Better Answer: Let's figure that out together.

The 24-hour day is divided into "fasting : eating" and could look like

12:12

14:10

16:8

18:6

OMAD (19:5, 20:4)

OPAD (23:1)

ADF (36:12, 40:8)

4:3

5:2

Time Restricted Eating

The minimum is 12:12, and common timeframes are 16:8 and 18:6. You may, however, choose ANY timeframe that works for your goals and your life.

OMAD

Many people mistakenly understand One Meal A Day to mean, "cramming all the food into one hour." Nothing could be further from the truth.

Take the components of One Meal – appetizer, salad, soup, roll, entrée, drink, dessert, tea – and spread it out over an enjoyable 2 to 5 hours. One Meal A Day, in a 19:5 timeframe is a satisfying and sustainable way to live.

After two months of experimenting, I settled into 20:4 OMAD as my fasting sweet spot. That is where I remain today, even after years in "maintenance" at my goal weight. I stick with this schedule because I can eat a lot in 4 hours, and fasting for 20 hours feels good to me!

OPAD

One Plate A Day could be a 23:1 schedule, and would be appropriate for people whose bodies do not feel deprived in any way by eating one satisfying meal in a very short eating window. This plan could be a useful short-term tool to break a stall, but *can* lower the metabolism over time. Eating in less than one hour is rarely a sustainable or satisfying way to live long term.

ADF

Alternate Day Fasting means switching back and forth, full fasting days ("Down Days") with full eating days ("Up Days"). This includes timing such as 36:12 and 40:8. ADF is an enticing approach for fasters who are committed to high levels of fat burning and autophagy, or who may be looking to reverse diseases such as type 2 diabetes.

Variations on a true ADF schedule include 4:3 (4 eating days & 3 full fasting days) and 5:2 (5 eating days & 2 full fasting days).

Some people choose to practice ADF short term, as I did in September 2018 to break my long five-month stall. Others are so delighted with this approach that they continue indefinitely. The idea of alternating fasting days with eating days can be extremely pleasurable and sustainable. Several days per week you may eat breakfast, lunch, *and* dinner!

The most important thing to remember regarding longer fasts (24+) is that you must schedule sufficient time to "reefed." Do not eat a quick meal, close your eating window, and start fasting again. This will tank your metabolism. Funnily enough, many people discover they are not hungry after a 36-hour fast, so you may need to eat a small amount of food, wait a few hours and eat more. My recommendation is that you always set aside 6 – 12 hours for eating after a long fast.

In order to contemplate an ideal eating window for you, first, write here the times that you currently eat. Include how often you have flavored snack-drinks, including creamy-sweet coffees.

Next, take a look at your wellness and weight goals. Add work, family, social life, and exercise regimen to your considerations.

What fasting:eating schedule would you like to start with?

Circle one of the following starting strategies:

Steady Start: 12 – 14 hours is fine. Rushing is not my style.

Stretch Start: 15 or 16 hours sounds like tough challenge.

Push Start: I'm going for it. 18 hours on day one.

Whatever schedule you choose to begin with is the *Perfect Start*. You may adjust it at any time, and you may slide the eating window around to match your plans.

Your clean fasting hours are healing hours, and the eating window is for nourishment and pleasure. Now that you know the value of fasting clean, and have a sense of a good starting schedule, let's EAT!

Eating: The Right Foods

This is where I inform you of the foods that you should eat, and foods that you should not eat.

Hint: I am not going to tell you what to eat.

Use these blank pages to make two lists:

- Foods and drinks that make me happy
- Foods and drinks that make me feel well, strong, and vibrant

Those are the foods you "should" eat. But... but... but? Yes, really.

The days of dieting deprivation are over! And, while you might adjust some of your foods to match your body's individual needs and sensitivities, that will come later. For now, in these first four weeks, eat the foods that you are looking forward to eating when your fast ends. Take the "Delay, Don't Deny" maxim to heart; fast clean and then you may eat delicious foods that make you happy.

Important

Please do not interpret this as permission to go overboard and gorge yourself with foods that make you feel bloated, sluggish, and ill.

If you ask ten different people about the best ways to eat, you will receive ten different answers. Theories on "clean eating" elicit a wide range of opinions and dogma. The only "right and best" foods are the foods that are "right and best" for *your* body.

I always remind people that the foods I ate when I was at my *ideal weight* were the same foods I ate when I *gained 50 pounds*. They were also the exact same foods I ate when I *lost 50 pounds* with intermittent fasting. The 50 pounds I gained had nothing to do with food, and everything to do with hormones. Similarly, the weight I lost had nothing to do with food, and everything to do with hormones.

Practice eating slowly, to satiety, until you are no longer hungry. In the beginning, it is common to eat ravenously out of fear – "I won't get to eat for SIXTEEN more hours!!!!" But, please, practice eating mindfully. Stop eating when you are no longer hungry. Your body *will* tell you, "enough."

Eat foods you love, and eat the foods that love you back.

Concerns & What to Expect

I shared this idea with a fasting friend recently, and she enthusiastically agreed, *"Dieting is easy to envision, yet difficult to execute. But, fasting is difficult to envision, yet easy to execute."*

I understand. It is impossible to envision what fasting will be like. Rest assured, clean fasting is *much* easier than you are imagining.

I want *nothing* to stand in the way of starting your first fast today, so let's tackle a few common concerns, and then get to fasting!

Loud Clamoring "Monkey Mind"

The EAT NOW conversation in your own head can be quite noisy in the first few days. It gets surprisingly quiet in short order. From time to time, the EAT NOW voice startles me, especially around the 16th hour of fasting. I laugh, order it to *shush*, and fast forward.

Waves of Hunger

Feelings of hunger arise from time to time in a wave, and then disappear. The wave does not get worse and worse. Breathe, have some icy cold mineral water, stay busy, and fast forward.

Growling Belly and Hunger Pangs

My favorite Gin Stephens line is, *"Hunger is not an emergency."* A noisy stomach might be embarrassing but we all have plenty of fuel on board. Instruct that rumbling engine to burn fat, and fast forward.

Feeling Poorly

I want to prepare you for three possible levels of struggle.

1. Clamoring noisy obnoxiousness mentioned above (Fast forward.)
2. Feeling a bit woozy (Put a few grains of high-quality salt *under* the tongue.)
3. Feeling shaky or unwell (Eat. Absolutely. 100%.)

Minerals/Electrolytes

Another important consideration is that when insulin is low, the kidneys dump magnesium and sodium. Magnesium is an electrolyte mineral, essential for hundreds of biochemical functions including cardiovascular, nerve, and muscle health.

You want to be prepared to replenish minerals by having an epsom salts bath, spraying magnesium on the bottoms of your feet, putting a few grains of high-quality salt under your tongue, drinking mineral water, or taking a magnesium capsule.

Feeling Cold

Your body is moving its energy towards the core while fat burning, thus leaving the extremities feeling chilly. This is great news. Layer up! You will warm up again after you eat.

Skin and Hair

Intermittent Fasting may play a part in short-term skin breakouts, itching or rashes, and hair loss. This is typically short-lived, and the skin and hair become even healthier.

Sleep

In the beginning, sleep may seem disrupted. However, it is common for intermittent fasters to feel more rested and refreshed in the morning, even if they are waking up from time to time or have more vivid dreams.

Digestion

The gut is repairing during your fasting hours, and during the adjustment phase you may experience changes in digestion. My advice is break your fast gently with a little fat and protein. This could be a hard-boiled egg, a few olives, perhaps a few bites of avocado. Ease in.

Changes in Menstrual Cycle

Intermittent Fasting *can* cause the cycle to alter temporarily. If you have irregular bleeding, please address this with your gynecologist. Also, you may feel ravenous in the days preceding your period. It is OK to extend your eating window and eat more during these days. Take wonderful care of yourself.

Closing the Eating Window at Night

It can be tough to resist "Captain Nightcap," as my friend, Mo, calls that sultry voice. The late night seductive plea for "more popcorn, finish the pint of ice cream, polish off the bottle" is predictable, and often results in "eating window creep."

If you suspect that slamming that window tight will be a challenge for you, schedule an earlier eating window – close it before 7PM — and repeat this same ritual every evening. Have a piece of expensive chocolate, sip a soothing herbal tea, then, BAM! Window Closed! Hit your fasting app "start fasting," brush your teeth, and enjoy an unflavored sparkling water in a fancy glass. Author, James Clear, calls this "Habit Stacking." Your cozy ritual will be locked in and Captain Nightcap will have no sway over you.

Write some ideas here about what some "Window Closing Rituals" could be for you:

What to Say to Others

We are accustomed to popping anything in our mouths that is offered to us, and we have learned to be uncomfortable in social settings unless we are eating. Now is the time to break those habits.

Here are a few ideas of what to say, and you *never* have to say, "I'm fasting."

"I'm not hungry right now."

"That looks delicious. [pop into ziplock] I'll enjoy it later!"

"I'm saving room for a big dinner."

"I am skipping lunch because it makes me sluggish and less productive. I want to feel awake at work!"

"Let's meet for a walk or coffee instead of lunch."

"It isn't time for me to eat yet, but, please, go right ahead."

"I already ate, but I would be happy to join you."

Add some more ideas here. What might you say to others when you tell them that you are not going to be eating right now?

Adjustment Phase Bingo

In Bingo, the goal is to cross off vertical, horizontal, and diagonal lines. Fill up as many as you can in your first four weeks! Heck, why not go for all sixteen? Let's play!

1	2	3	4
5	6	7	8
9	10	11	12
13	14	15	♥16

Cross off the corresponding box:

1 – While fasting, you use your old mealtimes to watch videos and listen to podcasts on Intermittent Fasting. Read one of the books from Laurie's list of resources.

2 – Plan your eating window so that you know what delicious foods you have to look forward to. Make "delaying" fun!

3 – Have a ziplock bag at the ready, so you can save treats for your window!

4 – Pause from your work, and rather than eating "al desko," treat yourself to a meal "al fresco." Take a break, make mealtime special.

5 – Download a fasting app so that you have a digital record of starting and stopping your fasting hours.

6 – Make window-closing fun! Create and practice your window-closing habits and rituals.

7 – Other than rushing to food for comfort, you have created a few other ways to soothe emotions and cope with stress.

8 – If you are tempted to break your fast early, imagine sirens and clanging bells in your head, "Insulin! Insulin! Insulin!" Nope, not yet. Fast forward!

9 – When growling ghrelin is clamoring for food, pretend the stomach noise is a fat-burning engine. Fast forward!

10 – You hit the 16-hour mark 3 days in a row! Cross off a bingo-box, and pour yourself a congratulatory sparkling water in a fancy glass!

11 – Do something sweet and kind for someone else. Fasting can be easier when the attention is off you.

12 – Feeling woozy for a second? Put a few grains of high-quality salt *under* your tongue.

13 – You told someone, "I'm not hungry right now," and have two other statements at the ready for when someone offers you food.

14 – While preparing food, you *almost* licked your fingers, but you didn't!!! Fast forward!

15 – You drank black coffee and didn't die.

16 – Freebie Square. YOU get to add one!

Measuring Progress

This is a starting point, so let's take a snapshot of where you are now. Use these pages as a log for *all* the possible ways to measure how you are doing along the way.

The scale does *not* have 100% of the vote here.

Circle the ones that you will be sure to do this week. It isn't fun, I know. Yet, you will be so glad you did it. I went down one clothing size in my first four weeks of fasting, but I forgot to take measurements. I really wish I had those simple numbers.

Goal Clothing

I recommend that you select two articles of clothing that you adore. The first is something that you can get on, but you would never go out of the house in it. Perhaps it zips, but you can't sit down. That's a good first one to select. And, the second is something that you can't get over your shoulders or up past your knees. But, you love that thing!

Hang these items for inspiration in a place that you can see them. Try them on incrementally just for fun.

Your two Goal Clothing items are:

1.

2.

Photos

Take pictures of your face, as well as your entire body, front, side, and back. You will be surprised how shocking it can be to see the back folds and squish disappearing. The face is important for a quick reference point as inflammation decreases, your eyes brighten, and your skin becomes smooth.

Measurements

At a minimum, measure your waist at your belly button. It is helpful, though to have a variety of other measures.

Date:	Date:
Neck:	Neck:
R Arm:	R Arm:
L Arm:	L Arm:
Chest:	Chest:
Waist:	Waist:
Hips:	Hips:
R Thigh:	R Thigh:
L Thigh:	L Thigh:
Date:	**Date:**
Neck:	Neck:
R Arm:	R Arm:
L Arm:	L Arm:
Chest:	Chest:
Waist:	Waist:
Hips:	Hips:
R Thigh:	R Thigh:
L Thigh:	L Thigh:

BMI

People shun Body Mass Index as an inaccurate way to determine "normal" or "healthy" weight. While there can be anomalies, it is a legitimate gauge for determining where you fall. Reaching the next level is inspiring.

Use google to determine your current BMI, and also indicate your goal number:

Now:

Goal:

Body Composition Scans

Two common ways to measure body composition are with machines that either use a very low dose of radiation (DEXA) or electrical impedance (InBody 570). If you find a fitness center or health clinic with one of these machines, confirm in advance that their machine will inform you of your "visceral fat" number.

I have found that the most important reason to spend money on these tests is to know exactly how much deadly fat is surrounding your organs. The body does *not* want that fat there, and research shows that visceral fat is the first to go. The body knows its priorities! If you decide to get a body composition scan done, watching the visceral fat diminish is highly motivating.

Be sure to keep the printouts of those reports here in this workbook.

Lab Work

Perhaps you have recently been to see your doctor and have fresh lab work. If not, consider making an appointment in the next month or so. It is important to know where you stand now, and compare with new numbers after you have been clean fasting for a year.

Tuck your recent reports in the back of this book, or jot down some of the important numbers here:

Weighing

We all have different relationships with the scale. We might view it as data only, a way to stay accountable. Yet, we often see it as a reflection of our worth, allowing it to determine our mood and sense of ourselves. Either way, it is difficult for us to fully understand that the scale will not tell us very much about the success of our intermittent fasting health journey.

The scale does not tell us the ways our body is healing.

The scale does not remind us that we are feeling less lethargic and more awake.

The scale does not remind us that we are not fixated on food all the time.

The scale does not inform us that our face and fingers are less puffy.

The scale does not remember that we are sleeping more soundly.

The scale does not let us know that we can climb stairs without being out of breath.

The scale does not show us that our belly is less bloated.

The scale does not indicate how much fat is coming off our organs.

The scale tells us one thing, our gravitational relationship to the floor.

An eye-opening thing about weight had me in giggles last year. Why do you *really* care about that number? "Unless your job is a horse racing jockey or a wrestler, WHY does that number matter?" screamed the comedian. Hmmmm, good question.

I won't tell you that the scale doesn't matter. I get it. I know it *does* matter. It's just that it is not the *only* data point.

Seeing the number go down over the first nine months *was* motivating for me. Some months it went down 2 pounds, other months 4-7 pounds. It kept inching, until it stopped. And, then, I was confused. I was 8 pounds from my goal weight. The scale stalled for 5 more months, spiraling up and down, round and round in the same 3-4 pound zone.

Goal weight is a calculated estimate, but we need to remember that it is arbitrary. Consider, the body is not on our schedule; it does not have the same timetables that we've manufactured. Sure, please set your goals and milestones, they can be motivating! Just don't forget; we made them up.

If you have a feeling that the number on the scale might not matter as much as you have thought it does, that, my friend, is the beginning of a uniquely personal and exciting discovery.

I am going to instruct and beg you to please NOT get on the scale for the first month of your intermittent fasting journey. During the first four weeks the body is adapting. You have never done this before, and it is adjusting! Do not subject yourself to surprising or demoralizing fluctuations on the scale.

I want you to stay motivated to continue, and discouragement is no fun. Therefore, my strong recommendation is to stay off it during these first 30 days. Please.

Try this. Weigh yourself for the next three days at the exact same time of day.

Write down those three numbers, add them up, divide by 3. That is your starting weight.

Day 1 weight:

Day 2 weight:

Day 3 weight:

Total:

/3 = Starting Weight:

Now, put the scale away.

When you get it out again in a month, you may decide that it is motivating to have the daily number.

The best way I have observed to have the scale work for you, is outlined by Gin Stephens in her first book. Weigh every day, add up the weekly total and divide by 7. That's your *average weight for the week*. Don't get stuck on the daily ups and downs. Only compare the weekly averages.

The following page has a grid for every week where you can track your progress. This is not a quick weight loss scheme. In my experience, the average over time for women might be one pound per week. I lost 51 pounds in 15 months, which averaged out to be approximately .85 pound per week. If that seems slow, consider that it is a lot quicker than it took gain the surplus fat.

Weight

Weekly Averages

Date		5-22-20
M	5-11-20	132.0
T	5-12-20	
W	5-13-20	130.5
T	5-14-20	130.5
F	5-15-20	
S	5-16-20	
S	5-17-20	
Add up the total =		
/7 for weekly avg =		
+up or -down =		

Date	
M	
T	
W	
T	
F	
S	
S	
Add up the total =	
/7 for weekly avg =	
+up or -down =	

Date	
M	
T	
W	
T	
F	
S	
S	
Add up the total =	
/7 for weekly avg =	
+up or -down =	

Date	
M	
T	
W	
T	
F	
S	
S	
Add up the total =	
/7 for weekly avg =	
+up or -down =	

Date	
M	
T	
W	
T	
F	
S	
S	
Add up the total =	
/7 for weekly avg =	
+up or -down =	

Date	
M	
T	
W	
T	
F	
S	
S	
Add up the total =	
/7 for weekly avg =	
+up or -down =	

Date	
M	
T	
W	
T	
F	
S	
S	
Add up the total =	
/7 for weekly avg =	
+up or -down =	

Date	
M	
T	
W	
T	
F	
S	
S	
Add up the total =	
/7 for weekly avg =	
+up or -down =	

Date	
M	
T	
W	
T	
F	
S	
S	
Add up the total =	
/7 for weekly avg =	
+up or -down =	

Date	
M	
T	
W	
T	
F	
S	
S	
Add up the total =	
/7 for weekly avg =	
+up or -down =	

Date	
M	
T	
W	
T	
F	
S	
S	
Add up the total =	
/7 for weekly avg =	
+up or -down =	

Date	
M	
T	
W	
T	
F	
S	
S	
Add up the total =	
/7 for weekly avg =	
+up or -down =	

Wins

Please list every good thing that happens along the way on your fasting journey. We call these, Non Scale Victories, NSVs. And, since this is a workbook dedicated to the celebration of you, let's celebrate everything!

-
-
-
-
-
-
-
-
-
-
-
-
-
-
-
-
-
-
-
-
-
-
-
-
-

Fast Forward

Let's Do This!

Let's not prolong this start any more —

PLAY BALL!

1. Stop eating today and note the time.

2. Set your fasting goal.

3. Drink plain water.

4. Sleep.

5. Wake up and drink a big glass of plain water.

6. Enjoy a cup of black coffee or tea.

7. Carry on with your day.

8. Open your eating window. (If you didn't make the fasting goal, no big deal!)

9. Eat and drink delicious foods until you are satisfied.

10. Close your eating window.

11. Repeat!

How to Use the Daily Log

1	DAY	DATE
FASTED	GOAL	ACHIEVED
WINDOW TIME	OPENED	CLOSED

- 1 2 3 4 5 6 7 8 9 10 +

FASTING

How I felt:

Tough times:

How I did it:

EATING

Opened Window with:

Next, I ate:

Eating pace:

Where I ate:

Closing Window ritual:

REFLECTIONS

Challenges:

One Good Thing:

- Write the Day of the Week and Date
- Enter the number of fasting hours you were aiming for, and what you actually achieved
- Circle a number 1-10 that represents how the day went for you. Overall, how challenging or fabulous was your fasting and eating today?
- Say more about how you felt while fasting
- If it got tough, document the time of day and # of hours fasted when it was hard. How long did the tough time last?
- Any tips for how you got through?
- What's the first thing you ate, and how did you feel?
- What did you eat next, and how did you feel?
- Was it "floodgates open," shove everything in? Or, did you eat at a leisurely pace?
- Did you eat in front of the computer or on the sofa? Were you in a restaurant, or at your kitchen table?
- What steps did you take to ensure "window closed" – "kitchen closed"?
- Take note of anything that was particularly difficult
- Write something good, and also add it to WINS list!
- A note to yourself, a pep talk, a tip… Don't Forget!

Week One

- Take your photos and measurements.
- Get out your calendar and plan your fasting and eating hours.
- Think of a few exciting meals that you can look forward to.
- Make no changes to food or exercise. Get out and walk, if you'd like to, but no intense gym sessions. Also, no "dieting," eat normal foods that you enjoy.
- Check Laurie's Corner for tips or inspiration. It's as if you're a fighter in the ring and I'm grabbing you by the shoulders and splashing water on your face.
- Go to the very back of this workbook and write a love letter to yourself that you will read in three months.
- Get out your tools. Tools? That's right. Got your plain water? Got your clock?

1　　　　　DAY Mon　　DATE 5/11/20

FASTED　　GOAL 20　　ACHIEVED 20½

WINDOW TIME　OPENED 3:30p　CLOSED 6:10p 8:30 pm

- 1 2 3 4 5 6 7 (8) 9 10 +

FASTING

How I felt: Fine - Back hurts

Tough times: No

How I did it: Just did

EATING

Opened Window with: Green greenhut cream salad Smoothie

Next, I ate: Spinach egg, chips Brussel sprouts, chicken Biscuit

Eating pace: Normal

Where I ate: TV / Living Room

Closing Window ritual: Decaf with milk & Splenda

REFLECTIONS

Challenges: Not eating junk or sugar

One Good Thing: Ate healthy, no sugar

2

DAY Tues DATE 5/12/20

FASTED GOAL 18 ACHIEVED
WINDOW TIME OPENED CLOSED

- 1 2 3 4 5 6 7 8 9 10 +

FASTING

How I felt:

Tough times:

How I did it:

EATING

Opened Window with:

Next, I ate:

Eating pace:

Where I ate:

Closing Window ritual:

REFLECTIONS

Challenges:

One Good Thing:

3

DAY Wed DATE 5-13-20

FASTED GOAL 18 ACHIEVED 21
WINDOW TIME OPENED 1:30 CLOSED 4pm

- 1 2 3 4 5 6 (7) 8 9 10 +

FASTING

How I felt:

Tough times:

How I did it:

EATING

Opened Window with:

Next, I ate:

Eating pace:

Where I ate:

Closing Window ritual:

REFLECTIONS

Challenges:

One Good Thing:

4 DAY 5-14-20 DATE Thurs

FASTED   GOAL 20   ACHIEVED

WINDOW TIME   OPENED   CLOSED

- 1 2 3 4 5 6 7 8 9 10 +

FASTING

How I felt:

Tough times:

How I did it:

EATING

Opened Window with:

Next, I ate:

Eating pace:

Where I ate:

Closing Window ritual:

REFLECTIONS

Challenges:

One Good Thing:

---

5 DAY   DATE

FASTED   GOAL   ACHIEVED

WINDOW TIME   OPENED   CLOSED

- 1 2 3 4 5 6 7 8 9 10 +

FASTING

How I felt:

Tough times:

How I did it:

EATING

Opened Window with:

Next, I ate:

Eating pace:

Where I ate:

Closing Window ritual:

REFLECTIONS

Challenges:

One Good Thing:

6	DAY	DATE	**7**	DAY	DATE
FASTED	GOAL	ACHIEVED	**FASTED**	GOAL	ACHIEVED
WINDOW TIME	OPENED	CLOSED	**WINDOW TIME**	OPENED	CLOSED

- 1 2 3 4 5 6 7 8 9 10 +   - 1 2 3 4 5 6 7 8 9 10 +

FASTING

How I felt:

Tough times:

How I did it:

EATING

Opened Window with:

Next, I ate:

Eating pace:

Where I ate:

Closing Window ritual:

REFLECTIONS

Challenges:

One Good Thing:

FASTING

How I felt:

Tough times:

How I did it:

EATING

Opened Window with:

Next, I ate:

Eating pace:

Where I ate:

Closing Window ritual:

REFLECTIONS

Challenges:

One Good Thing:

Week One

Reflections

List what surprised you this week.

What are some questions that you have?

Double-check, make absolutely certain you are fasting clean.

List some of the challenges you faced in this first week.

Laurie's Corner

Be serious. Be disciplined.
Do the work.

Oh! And, don't forget to
eat delicious food!

Week Two

The Push

- ❯ If you are going for the Steady Start, increase your fasting by 15 minutes every day. We are aiming for 16:8 within the next week.

- ❯ Stretch Start ladies, you have most likely reached 16:8 already.

- ❯ Push Start team, your fasting hours may vary every day because 18 hours out of the gate is tough. Do not be upset if some days are 16 and other days are 18.

- ❯ Between weeks 2 and 3, you may go through a rough patch for a few days. The glycogen stores might be nearing depletion, and you could be edgier and moodier than normal. This will pass.

- ❯ If you have a question if a tea, water, coffee or supplement is allowed during the clean fasting hours, read the Ingredients closely, and compare to the Yes column of the Clean Fast Chart.

- ❯ Remember to flip back and cross off those Fasting Bingo boxes!

- ❯ Is it too late to remind you it is OK to brush your teeth? Sure, it's minty and flavorful, but brush, rinse, and carry-on.

- ❯ Same goes for communion at church. Fulfill your religious and spiritual practices.

8   DAY   DATE
FASTED   GOAL   ACHIEVED
WINDOW TIME   OPENED   CLOSED

- 1 2 3 4 5 6 7 8 9 10 +

FASTING

How I felt:

Tough times:

How I did it:

EATING

Opened Window with:

Next, I ate:

Eating pace:

Where I ate:

Closing Window ritual:

REFLECTIONS

Challenges:

One Good Thing:

9	DAY	DATE		**10**	DAY	DATE
FASTED	GOAL	ACHIEVED		**FASTED**	GOAL	ACHIEVED
WINDOW TIME	OPENED	CLOSED		**WINDOW TIME**	OPENED	CLOSED

- 1 2 3 4 5 6 7 8 9 10 +   - 1 2 3 4 5 6 7 8 9 10 +

FASTING

How I felt:

Tough times:

How I did it:

EATING

Opened Window with:

Next, I ate:

Eating pace:

Where I ate:

Closing Window ritual:

REFLECTIONS

Challenges:

One Good Thing:

FASTING

How I felt:

Tough times:

How I did it:

EATING

Opened Window with:

Next, I ate:

Eating pace:

Where I ate:

Closing Window ritual:

REFLECTIONS

Challenges:

One Good Thing:

11 DAY   DATE   **12** DAY   DATE
FASTED GOAL ACHIEVED   **FASTED** GOAL ACHIEVED
WINDOW TIME OPENED CLOSED   **WINDOW TIME** OPENED CLOSED

- 1 2 3 4 5 6 7 8 9 10 +   - 1 2 3 4 5 6 7 8 9 10 +

FASTING

How I felt:

Tough times:

How I did it:

EATING

Opened Window with:

Next, I ate:

Eating pace:

Where I ate:

Closing Window ritual:

REFLECTIONS

Challenges:

One Good Thing:

FASTING

How I felt:

Tough times:

How I did it:

EATING

Opened Window with:

Next, I ate:

Eating pace:

Where I ate:

Closing Window ritual:

REFLECTIONS

Challenges:

One Good Thing:

13   DAY   DATE

FASTED   GOAL   ACHIEVED

WINDOW TIME   OPENED   CLOSED

- 1   2   3   4   5   6   7   8   9   10 +

FASTING

How I felt:

Tough times:

How I did it:

EATING

Opened Window with:

Next, I ate:

Eating pace:

Where I ate:

Closing Window ritual:

REFLECTIONS

Challenges:

One Good Thing:

---

14   DAY   DATE

FASTED   GOAL   ACHIEVED

WINDOW TIME   OPENED   CLOSED

- 1   2   3   4   5   6   7   8   9   10 +

FASTING

How I felt:

Tough times:

How I did it:

EATING

Opened Window with:

Next, I ate:

Eating pace:

Where I ate:

Closing Window ritual:

REFLECTIONS

Challenges:

One Good Thing:

Week Two

Reflections

Even if the best you can say is you "have reduced bloat and blah," say it!

What is something small you can identify and be grateful for?

And, if you are still discovering, say that here. "I am still discovering."

Hang in there, friend. Remind yourself of what went well today.

Have you spoken with anyone about your new fasting regimen? How did that go?

What challenges have you had scheduling and preparing your meals? What adjustments can you make regarding planning?

Laurie's Corner

Get out your calendar and pencil in all your fasts and eating windows for the week. What will you eat first?

Week Three

The Bold Stretch

- This week you will try your first 20 hour fast.

- This bold stretch builds confidence.

- After achieving your personal best, going back to 16 or 18 hours won't seem that difficult.

- Trying a 20 hour fast from Sunday to Monday is often a good idea. Close the eating window around 4PM on Sunday, and fast until noon on Monday.

- Have your mineral water and high-quality salt on hand.

- Stay busy!

- Know what delicious foods you will be enjoying at noon, and ease in.

15   DAY   DATE

FASTED   GOAL   ACHIEVED

WINDOW TIME   OPENED   CLOSED

- 1 2 3 4 5 6 7 8 9 10 +

FASTING

How I felt:

Tough times:

How I did it:

EATING

Opened Window with:

Next, I ate:

Eating pace:

Where I ate:

Closing Window ritual:

REFLECTIONS

Challenges:

One Good Thing:

16	DAY	DATE	**17**	DAY	DATE
FASTED	GOAL	ACHIEVED	**FASTED**	GOAL	ACHIEVED
WINDOW TIME	OPENED	CLOSED	**WINDOW TIME**	OPENED	CLOSED

- 1 2 3 4 5 6 7 8 9 10 +   - 1 2 3 4 5 6 7 8 9 10 +

FASTING

How I felt:

Tough times:

How I did it:

EATING

Opened Window with:

Next, I ate:

Eating pace:

Where I ate:

Closing Window ritual:

REFLECTIONS

Challenges:

One Good Thing:

FASTING

How I felt:

Tough times:

How I did it:

EATING

Opened Window with:

Next, I ate:

Eating pace:

Where I ate:

Closing Window ritual:

REFLECTIONS

Challenges:

One Good Thing:

18	DAY	DATE	**19**	DAY	DATE
FASTED	GOAL	ACHIEVED	**FASTED**	GOAL	ACHIEVED
WINDOW TIME	OPENED	CLOSED	**WINDOW TIME**	OPENED	CLOSED

- 1 2 3 4 5 6 7 8 9 10 +   - 1 2 3 4 5 6 7 8 9 10 +

FASTING

How I felt:

Tough times:

How I did it:

EATING

Opened Window with:

Next, I ate:

Eating pace:

Where I ate:

Closing Window ritual:

REFLECTIONS

Challenges:

One Good Thing:

FASTING

How I felt:

Tough times:

How I did it:

EATING

Opened Window with:

Next, I ate:

Eating pace:

Where I ate:

Closing Window ritual:

REFLECTIONS

Challenges:

One Good Thing:

20   DAY   DATE

FASTED   GOAL   ACHIEVED

WINDOW TIME   OPENED   CLOSED

- 1 2 3 4 5 6 7 8 9 10 +

FASTING

How I felt:

Tough times:

How I did it:

EATING

Opened Window with:

Next, I ate:

Eating pace:

Where I ate:

Closing Window ritual:

REFLECTIONS

Challenges:

One Good Thing:

---

21   DAY   DATE

FASTED   GOAL   ACHIEVED

WINDOW TIME   OPENED   CLOSED

- 1 2 3 4 5 6 7 8 9 10 +

FASTING

How I felt:

Tough times:

How I did it:

EATING

Opened Window with:

Next, I ate:

Eating pace:

Where I ate:

Closing Window ritual:

REFLECTIONS

Challenges:

One Good Thing:

Week Three

Reflections

Share here what the 20 hour fast was like for you. Jot down everything you can remember.

What non-food rewards are you giving yourself to celebrate?

Notice how certain foods are making you feel. Are you getting sleepy after you eat? What foods are working, or not working to open your eating window?

Consider, you are either "fed or fasted," as ole' Butter Bob Briggs states so profoundly in one of his videos. The idea of eating certain foods in order to lose weight is utterly absurd. Just think about it. What are the foods we should eat to lose weight? Fast clean and long to burn fat, and then select foods that make you happy.

What are you seeing already about the benefits of clean fasting?

Laurie's Corner

You knocked it out of the park with that Personal Best fast. We aren't aiming for perfection, we are stretching! Well done.

Week Four

Noticing-Noticing-Noticing

- Notice if your energy feels even throughout the day
- Notice what fasting hours feel right
- Notice what foods make you feel awful
- Notice the foods that make you feel well
- Notice when the body is telling you to stop eating
- Notice your thoughts about fasting
- Notice how your feeling during times of the day when you used to feel sluggish
- Notice what you love about this
- Notice if you are enjoying the discovery and the challenge

22   DAY   DATE

FASTED   GOAL   ACHIEVED

WINDOW TIME   OPENED   CLOSED

- 1   2   3   4   5   6   7   8   9   10 +

FASTING

How I felt:

Tough times:

How I did it:

EATING

Opened Window with:

Next, I ate:

Eating pace:

Where I ate:

Closing Window ritual:

REFLECTIONS

Challenges:

One Good Thing:

23 DAY DATE
FASTED GOAL ACHIEVED
WINDOW TIME OPENED CLOSED

- 1 2 3 4 5 6 7 8 9 10 +

FASTING

How I felt:

Tough times:

How I did it:

EATING

Opened Window with:

Next, I ate:

Eating pace:

Where I ate:

Closing Window ritual:

REFLECTIONS

Challenges:

One Good Thing:

---

24 DAY DATE
FASTED GOAL ACHIEVED
WINDOW TIME OPENED CLOSED

- 1 2 3 4 5 6 7 8 9 10 +

FASTING

How I felt:

Tough times:

How I did it:

EATING

Opened Window with:

Next, I ate:

Eating pace:

Where I ate:

Closing Window ritual:

REFLECTIONS

Challenges:

One Good Thing:

25   DAY   DATE

FASTED   GOAL   ACHIEVED

WINDOW TIME   OPENED   CLOSED

- 1   2   3   4   5   6   7   8   9   10 +

FASTING

How I felt:

Tough times:

How I did it:

EATING

Opened Window with:

Next, I ate:

Eating pace:

Where I ate:

Closing Window ritual:

REFLECTIONS

Challenges:

One Good Thing:

---

26   DAY   DATE

FASTED   GOAL   ACHIEVED

WINDOW TIME   OPENED   CLOSED

- 1   2   3   4   5   6   7   8   9   10 +

FASTING

How I felt:

Tough times:

How I did it:

EATING

Opened Window with:

Next, I ate:

Eating pace:

Where I ate:

Closing Window ritual:

REFLECTIONS

Challenges:

One Good Thing:

27 DAY DATE
FASTED GOAL ACHIEVED
WINDOW TIME OPENED CLOSED

- 1 2 3 4 5 6 7 8 9 10 +

FASTING

How I felt:

Tough times:

How I did it:

EATING

Opened Window with:

Next, I ate:

Eating pace:

Where I ate:

Closing Window ritual:

REFLECTIONS

Challenges:

One Good Thing:

28 DAY DATE
FASTED GOAL ACHIEVED
WINDOW TIME OPENED CLOSED

- 1 2 3 4 5 6 7 8 9 10 +

FASTING

How I felt:

Tough times:

How I did it:

EATING

Opened Window with:

Next, I ate:

Eating pace:

Where I ate:

Closing Window ritual:

REFLECTIONS

Challenges:

One Good Thing:

Week Four

Reflections

Rather than being frustrated with the unknowns, could you approach it as a science experiment and simply observe? Isn't that interesting?

If you allowed it to be fascinating, what could you discern and conclude?

In moments of doubt, what has inspired you to keep going? What are you saying to yourself?

Is there someone in your life who has endured insurmountable challenges? Call you call upon them and use them for inspiration? Who can you think of, and what inspires you?

Laurie's Corner

Many years back a friend barely survived a tragic accident. Their family motto was, "Murphy's Don't Quit." At times of personal struggle, I often think of them, and I pretend that I am a Murphy.

Settling Into My Groove!

Week Five

My Sweetspot

- Notice if you are getting a funny taste in your mouth (ketosis)
- Notice if foods you used to like now taste terrible to you (appetite correction)
- Notice if you are interested in foods you haven't thought of in a while
- Notice if you aren't too hungry one day, and then extra hungry the next day
- Notice if you are agitated about slow results, or elated if you have speedy results
- Notice if you handled a challenging situation more peacefully than you may have in the past
- Review the Fasting: Schedules section and ponder what regimen you might like to settle in on
- I recommend that you attempt 19:5 for a week, just to see what it feels like to get in that extra fat-burning, and to eat well in a five-hour eating window.

29   DAY   DATE

FASTED   GOAL   ACHIEVED

WINDOW TIME   OPENED   CLOSED

- 1   2   3   4   5   6   7   8   9   10 +

FASTING

How I felt:

Tough times:

How I did it:

EATING

Opened Window with:

Next, I ate:

Eating pace:

Where I ate:

Closing Window ritual:

REFLECTIONS

Challenges:

One Good Thing:

30	DAY	DATE	**31**	DAY	DATE
FASTED	GOAL	ACHIEVED	**FASTED**	GOAL	ACHIEVED
WINDOW TIME	OPENED	CLOSED	**WINDOW TIME**	OPENED	CLOSED

- 1 2 3 4 5 6 7 8 9 10 +   - 1 2 3 4 5 6 7 8 9 10 +

FASTING

How I felt:

Tough times:

How I did it:

EATING

Opened Window with:

Next, I ate:

Eating pace:

Where I ate:

Closing Window ritual:

REFLECTIONS

Challenges:

One Good Thing:

FASTING

How I felt:

Tough times:

How I did it:

EATING

Opened Window with:

Next, I ate:

Eating pace:

Where I ate:

Closing Window ritual:

REFLECTIONS

Challenges:

One Good Thing:

32	DAY	DATE	**33**	DAY	DATE
FASTED	GOAL	ACHIEVED	**FASTED**	GOAL	ACHIEVED
WINDOW TIME	OPENED	CLOSED	**WINDOW TIME**	OPENED	CLOSED

- 1 2 3 4 5 6 7 8 9 10 +   - 1 2 3 4 5 6 7 8 9 10 +

FASTING

How I felt:

Tough times:

How I did it:

EATING

Opened Window with:

Next, I ate:

Eating pace:

Where I ate:

Closing Window ritual:

REFLECTIONS

Challenges:

One Good Thing:

FASTING

How I felt:

Tough times:

How I did it:

EATING

Opened Window with:

Next, I ate:

Eating pace:

Where I ate:

Closing Window ritual:

REFLECTIONS

Challenges:

One Good Thing:

34	DAY	DATE	**35**	DAY	DATE
FASTED	GOAL	ACHIEVED	**FASTED**	GOAL	ACHIEVED
WINDOW TIME	OPENED	CLOSED	**WINDOW TIME**	OPENED	CLOSED

- 1 2 3 4 5 6 7 8 9 10 +   - 1 2 3 4 5 6 7 8 9 10 +

FASTING

How I felt:

Tough times:

How I did it:

EATING

Opened Window with:

Next, I ate:

Eating pace:

Where I ate:

Closing Window ritual:

REFLECTIONS

Challenges:

One Good Thing:

FASTING

How I felt:

Tough times:

How I did it:

EATING

Opened Window with:

Next, I ate:

Eating pace:

Where I ate:

Closing Window ritual:

REFLECTIONS

Challenges:

One Good Thing:

Week Five

Reflections

Are there ways you are developing a newfound respect for your body? What are some of the things you respect about it? What could you be in awe of?

Is there someone you could take someone under your wing and share with them about intermittent fasting? Who could benefit from this practice?

The signs of Appetite Correction are definitely kicking in. What do you see:

What new and uplifting rituals and practices are you already putting in place?

Laurie's Corner

Give yourself a high five and a happy dance. This is going GREAT!

Week Six

Hitting My Stride

- Have you had any opportunities to travel, go to events or parties, or shake up your fasting routine? Remember, it is flexible!

- You might be cruising along with fasting and suddenly get a cold or seasonal allergies kick in. Use your best judgment regarding when to fast. There is no problem setting your fasting regimen aside for a few days.

- If you begin to develop any health challenges, many people automatically assume that "fasting caused it!" Every new issue that arises in the body is not caused by fasting. Use fasting as your foundation for health, and when necessary, bring your health issues to your physician. Always inform your healthcare practitioners that you are practicing a daily clean fasting regimen.

- Scan your body top to bottom and notice anything that is "healing."

- Body shape changes while fasting even when the scale doesn't budge.

36   DAY   DATE

FASTED   GOAL   ACHIEVED

WINDOW TIME   OPENED   CLOSED

- 1 2 3 4 5 6 7 8 9 10 +

FASTING

How I felt:

Tough times:

How I did it:

EATING

Opened Window with:

Next, I ate:

Eating pace:

Where I ate:

Closing Window ritual:

REFLECTIONS

Challenges:

One Good Thing:

37	DAY	DATE	**38**	DAY	DATE
FASTED	GOAL	ACHIEVED	**FASTED**	GOAL	ACHIEVED
WINDOW TIME	OPENED	CLOSED	**WINDOW TIME**	OPENED	CLOSED

- 1 2 3 4 5 6 7 8 9 10 +   - 1 2 3 4 5 6 7 8 9 10 +

FASTING

How I felt:

Tough times:

How I did it:

EATING

Opened Window with:

Next, I ate:

Eating pace:

Where I ate:

Closing Window ritual:

REFLECTIONS

Challenges:

One Good Thing:

FASTING

How I felt:

Tough times:

How I did it:

EATING

Opened Window with:

Next, I ate:

Eating pace:

Where I ate:

Closing Window ritual:

REFLECTIONS

Challenges:

One Good Thing:

39   DAY   DATE
FASTED   GOAL   ACHIEVED
WINDOW TIME   OPENED   CLOSED

- 1   2   3   4   5   6   7   8   9   10 +

FASTING

How I felt:

Tough times:

How I did it:

EATING

Opened Window with:

Next, I ate:

Eating pace:

Where I ate:

Closing Window ritual:

REFLECTIONS

Challenges:

One Good Thing:

40   DAY   DATE
FASTED   GOAL   ACHIEVED
WINDOW TIME   OPENED   CLOSED

- 1   2   3   4   5   6   7   8   9   10 +

FASTING

How I felt:

Tough times:

How I did it:

EATING

Opened Window with:

Next, I ate:

Eating pace:

Where I ate:

Closing Window ritual:

REFLECTIONS

Challenges:

One Good Thing:

41 DAY DATE   **42** DAY DATE
FASTED GOAL ACHIEVED   **FASTED** GOAL ACHIEVED
WINDOW TIME OPENED CLOSED   **WINDOW TIME** OPENED CLOSED

- 1 2 3 4 5 6 7 8 9 10 +   - 1 2 3 4 5 6 7 8 9 10 +

FASTING

How I felt:

Tough times:

How I did it:

EATING

Opened Window with:

Next, I ate:

Eating pace:

Where I ate:

Closing Window ritual:

REFLECTIONS

Challenges:

One Good Thing:

FASTING

How I felt:

Tough times:

How I did it:

EATING

Opened Window with:

Next, I ate:

Eating pace:

Where I ate:

Closing Window ritual:

REFLECTIONS

Challenges:

One Good Thing:

Week Six

Reflections

Sometimes people feel at this point that it is hard, they could be bored, they keep falling off, can't do it, they are alone in this. It is a general malaise that feels out of our control. If you have hit boredom, frustration, or resentment, write more about that here.

When you feel as if you have hit your fasting sweet spot, or are in your fasting groove, describe that here.

Laurie's Corner

The ups and downs are *all* part of it. Observe those experiences and show yourself grace. Big hugs.

Week Seven

Taking Stock

- Up your movement, but don't over-do it. If intense exercise adds to your stress load, don't push it!

- If you love to exercise and your body is crying out for more movement, try out exercising while fasting! At this point, your body is burning fat for energy, and working out is a great idea.

- Really use this week to look at how far you have come regarding your fasting hours, foods, sleep, and mood.

- Dig around on the internet for the latest research on intermittent fasting.

- Go to the WINS list and fill out every good thing that has happened over the last few days

---

43   DAY   DATE

FASTED   GOAL   ACHIEVED

WINDOW TIME   OPENED   CLOSED

- 1   2   3   4   5   6   7   8   9   10 +

FASTING

How I felt:

Tough times:

How I did it:

EATING

Opened Window with:

Next, I ate:

Eating pace:

Where I ate:

Closing Window ritual:

REFLECTIONS

Challenges:

One Good Thing:

44		DAY	DATE	**45**		DAY	DATE
FASTED		GOAL	ACHIEVED	**FASTED**		GOAL	ACHIEVED
WINDOW TIME		OPENED	CLOSED	**WINDOW TIME**		OPENED	CLOSED

- 1 2 3 4 5 6 7 8 9 10 +   - 1 2 3 4 5 6 7 8 9 10 +

FASTING

How I felt:

Tough times:

How I did it:

EATING

Opened Window with:

Next, I ate:

Eating pace:

Where I ate:

Closing Window ritual:

REFLECTIONS

Challenges:

One Good Thing:

FASTING

How I felt:

Tough times:

How I did it:

EATING

Opened Window with:

Next, I ate:

Eating pace:

Where I ate:

Closing Window ritual:

REFLECTIONS

Challenges:

One Good Thing:

46 DAY DATE
FASTED GOAL ACHIEVED
WINDOW TIME OPENED CLOSED

- 1 2 3 4 5 6 7 8 9 10 +

FASTING

How I felt:

Tough times:

How I did it:

EATING

Opened Window with:

Next, I ate:

Eating pace:

Where I ate:

Closing Window ritual:

REFLECTIONS

Challenges:

One Good Thing:

---

47 DAY DATE
FASTED GOAL ACHIEVED
WINDOW TIME OPENED CLOSED

- 1 2 3 4 5 6 7 8 9 10 +

FASTING

How I felt:

Tough times:

How I did it:

EATING

Opened Window with:

Next, I ate:

Eating pace:

Where I ate:

Closing Window ritual:

REFLECTIONS

Challenges:

One Good Thing:

48   DAY   DATE

FASTED   GOAL   ACHIEVED

WINDOW TIME   OPENED   CLOSED

- 1 2 3 4 5 6 7 8 9 10 +

FASTING

How I felt:

Tough times:

How I did it:

EATING

Opened Window with:

Next, I ate:

Eating pace:

Where I ate:

Closing Window ritual:

REFLECTIONS

Challenges:

One Good Thing:

---

49   DAY   DATE

FASTED   GOAL   ACHIEVED

WINDOW TIME   OPENED   CLOSED

- 1 2 3 4 5 6 7 8 9 10 +

FASTING

How I felt:

Tough times:

How I did it:

EATING

Opened Window with:

Next, I ate:

Eating pace:

Where I ate:

Closing Window ritual:

REFLECTIONS

Challenges:

One Good Thing:

Week Seven

Reflections

If you have started any sentences with, "I'm so mad at myself," please know, I am not mad at you. I can probably see ten amazing things you've done, and I want you to see them too. Set aside frustration, and tell me something amazing.

If someone asked you to tell them how to start Intermittent Fasting, what would you tell them? How should they get started? And, what are your top tips?

Laurie's Corner

Remember, this journey is yours alone. It does not matter at all what is happening on the scale for someone else. This is ALL YOU! And, I believe in you.

Week Eight

A New Stretch

- Have you been wondering, Why am I doing this again? How about... Neuroplasticity! For the growth and nurturing of new brain cells and connections! Daily detox is a requirement! Clean out the debris in our cells.

- Read a book off Laurie's Resources list in the back

- Listen to Gin Stephen's podcast interviews, "Intermittent Fasting Stories." I'm episode #4!

- Start pondering about your fasting mantra. What is it you say to yourself to get pumped up and over a hump?

- Do you like the time of your eating window? If you would like to move it around this week, give that a try!

- Schedule one Stretch Day every week. The Stretch Day could be 20, 24, or even 36 hours.

- Try on those Goal Jeans and take new measurements

---

50   DAY   DATE

FASTED   GOAL   ACHIEVED

WINDOW TIME   OPENED   CLOSED

- 1 2 3 4 5 6 7 8 9 10 +

FASTING

How I felt:

Tough times:

How I did it:

EATING

Opened Window with:

Next, I ate:

Eating pace:

Where I ate:

Closing Window ritual:

REFLECTIONS

Challenges:

One Good Thing:

51	DAY	DATE	**52**	DAY	DATE
FASTED	GOAL	ACHIEVED	**FASTED**	GOAL	ACHIEVED
WINDOW TIME	OPENED	CLOSED	**WINDOW TIME**	OPENED	CLOSED

- 1 2 3 4 5 6 7 8 9 10 +   - 1 2 3 4 5 6 7 8 9 10 +

FASTING

How I felt:

Tough times:

How I did it:

EATING

Opened Window with:

Next, I ate:

Eating pace:

Where I ate:

Closing Window ritual:

REFLECTIONS

Challenges:

One Good Thing:

FASTING

How I felt:

Tough times:

How I did it:

EATING

Opened Window with:

Next, I ate:

Eating pace:

Where I ate:

Closing Window ritual:

REFLECTIONS

Challenges:

One Good Thing:

53	DAY	DATE
FASTED	GOAL	ACHIEVED
WINDOW TIME	OPENED	CLOSED

- 1 2 3 4 5 6 7 8 9 10 +

FASTING

How I felt:

Tough times:

How I did it:

EATING

Opened Window with:

Next, I ate:

Eating pace:

Where I ate:

Closing Window ritual:

REFLECTIONS

Challenges:

One Good Thing:

54	DAY	DATE
FASTED	GOAL	ACHIEVED
WINDOW TIME	OPENED	CLOSED

- 1 2 3 4 5 6 7 8 9 10 +

FASTING

How I felt:

Tough times:

How I did it:

EATING

Opened Window with:

Next, I ate:

Eating pace:

Where I ate:

Closing Window ritual:

REFLECTIONS

Challenges:

One Good Thing:

55 DAY DATE **56** DAY DATE
FASTED GOAL ACHIEVED **FASTED** GOAL ACHIEVED
WINDOW TIME OPENED CLOSED **WINDOW TIME** OPENED CLOSED

- 1 2 3 4 5 6 7 8 9 10 +   - 1 2 3 4 5 6 7 8 9 10 +

FASTING

How I felt:

Tough times:

How I did it:

EATING

Opened Window with:

Next, I ate:

Eating pace:

Where I ate:

Closing Window ritual:

REFLECTIONS

Challenges:

One Good Thing:

FASTING

How I felt:

Tough times:

How I did it:

EATING

Opened Window with:

Next, I ate:

Eating pace:

Where I ate:

Closing Window ritual:

REFLECTIONS

Challenges:

One Good Thing:

Week Eight

Reflections

Forget about the number on the scale. Think, what is it about being strong and lean that is desireable? If you could forget about the scale, what do you want your body to be able to do?

What do you want your body to look like and feel like?

Are you feeling closer to that measure?

In what ways do you hear and see that your fasting practice is being directed by your inner authority? Are you less interested external directions, and more in tuned with what your body is telling you?

Write a bit about that:

Laurie's Corner

You deserve the very best. Only choose foods that are "Window Worthy"!!

Great Way to Live

Week Nine

My Fasting Mantra

- ❯ Look for ways to make tiny 1 degree shifts. Small steps aggregate into major shifts and healing.
- ❯ It takes 28 - 40 days for a new habit to be locked in.
- ❯ Notice what you say to yourself to pump yourself up
- ❯ Flip back and add more WINS to the NSV list
- ❯ Notice if any foods are presenting challenges
- ❯ My friend, Kim says to "keep fasting boring and joyful." Could you try that on?

57	DAY	DATE
FASTED	GOAL	ACHIEVED
WINDOW TIME	OPENED	CLOSED

- 1 2 3 4 5 6 7 8 9 10 +

FASTING

How I felt:

Tough times:

How I did it:

EATING

Opened Window with:

Next, I ate:

Eating pace:

Where I ate:

Closing Window ritual:

REFLECTIONS

Challenges:

One Good Thing:

58	DAY	DATE		**59**	DAY	DATE
FASTED	GOAL	ACHIEVED		**FASTED**	GOAL	ACHIEVED
WINDOW TIME	OPENED	CLOSED		**WINDOW TIME**	OPENED	CLOSED

- 1 2 3 4 5 6 7 8 9 10 +   - 1 2 3 4 5 6 7 8 9 10 +

FASTING

How I felt:

Tough times:

How I did it:

EATING

Opened Window with:

Next, I ate:

Eating pace:

Where I ate:

Closing Window ritual:

REFLECTIONS

Challenges:

One Good Thing:

FASTING

How I felt:

Tough times:

How I did it:

EATING

Opened Window with:

Next, I ate:

Eating pace:

Where I ate:

Closing Window ritual:

REFLECTIONS

Challenges:

One Good Thing:

60   DAY   DATE
FASTED   GOAL   ACHIEVED
WINDOW TIME   OPENED   CLOSED

- 1 2 3 4 5 6 7 8 9 10 +

FASTING

How I felt:

Tough times:

How I did it:

EATING

Opened Window with:

Next, I ate:

Eating pace:

Where I ate:

Closing Window ritual:

REFLECTIONS

Challenges:

One Good Thing:

---

61   DAY   DATE
FASTED   GOAL   ACHIEVED
WINDOW TIME   OPENED   CLOSED

- 1 2 3 4 5 6 7 8 9 10 +

FASTING

How I felt:

Tough times:

How I did it:

EATING

Opened Window with:

Next, I ate:

Eating pace:

Where I ate:

Closing Window ritual:

REFLECTIONS

Challenges:

One Good Thing:

62   DAY   DATE

FASTED   GOAL   ACHIEVED

WINDOW TIME   OPENED   CLOSED

- 1 2 3 4 5 6 7 8 9 10 +

FASTING

How I felt:

Tough times:

How I did it:

EATING

Opened Window with:

Next, I ate:

Eating pace:

Where I ate:

Closing Window ritual:

REFLECTIONS

Challenges:

One Good Thing:

---

63   DAY   DATE

FASTED   GOAL   ACHIEVED

WINDOW TIME   OPENED   CLOSED

- 1 2 3 4 5 6 7 8 9 10 +

FASTING

How I felt:

Tough times:

How I did it:

EATING

Opened Window with:

Next, I ate:

Eating pace:

Where I ate:

Closing Window ritual:

REFLECTIONS

Challenges:

One Good Thing:

Week Nine

Reflections

What are you grateful for?

List ALL of the possible Mantras that you could own as *the* thing that keeps you going.

Here are some suggestions:

"Delay, Don't Deny"

"Fasting is a gift"

"My Fasting hours are my healing hours"

"My body is AMAZING"

"Trust the Process"

"I love tweaking and tinkering"

"My body is in the driver's seat"

"My body isn't on my timeline"

"Fasting clean is good for me"

"I am a healthy person"

"This is unbelievable freedom"

"I am enjoying my life and my choices"

Keep writing...

Laurie's Corner

I love how you are owning this.
You inspire me.

Week Ten

Considering My Future

- Create a local meet-up for Intermittent Fasters

- At our age, some common things that can cause pronounced imbalance with our hormones are:

  - Toxins in our environment, food, and skincare products
  - Ultra-processed factory-made foods
  - Chronic inflammation
  - Mitochondria imbalance

- Consider seeking out a deeper understanding of other aspects of our daily living that pose health risks

- When I say, "Listen to your body," you may understand what I mean now. The thoughts come as a very quiet voice, like, "Maybe you can run again," or, "Spinach sounds delicious," or, "You haven't made an omelette in a while." Pay attention to those types of calm and peaceful communications.

64   DAY   DATE

FASTED   GOAL   ACHIEVED

WINDOW TIME   OPENED   CLOSED

- 1   2   3   4   5   6   7   8   9   10 +

FASTING

How I felt:

Tough times:

How I did it:

EATING

Opened Window with:

Next, I ate:

Eating pace:

Where I ate:

Closing Window ritual:

REFLECTIONS

Challenges:

One Good Thing:

65　　　DAY　　　DATE　　　　**66**　　　DAY　　　DATE

FASTED　　GOAL　　ACHIEVED　　**FASTED**　　GOAL　　ACHIEVED

WINDOW TIME　　OPENED　　CLOSED　　**WINDOW TIME**　　OPENED　　CLOSED

- 1　2　3　4　5　6　7　8　9　10 +　　　　- 1　2　3　4　5　6　7　8　9　10 +

FASTING

How I felt:

Tough times:

How I did it:

EATING

Opened Window with:

Next, I ate:

Eating pace:

Where I ate:

Closing Window ritual:

REFLECTIONS

Challenges:

One Good Thing:

FASTING

How I felt:

Tough times:

How I did it:

EATING

Opened Window with:

Next, I ate:

Eating pace:

Where I ate:

Closing Window ritual:

REFLECTIONS

Challenges:

One Good Thing:

67	DAY	DATE	**68**	DAY	DATE
FASTED	GOAL	ACHIEVED	**FASTED**	GOAL	ACHIEVED
WINDOW TIME	OPENED	CLOSED	**WINDOW TIME**	OPENED	CLOSED

- 1 2 3 4 5 6 7 8 9 10 +   - 1 2 3 4 5 6 7 8 9 10 +

FASTING

How I felt:

Tough times:

How I did it:

EATING

Opened Window with:

Next, I ate:

Eating pace:

Where I ate:

Closing Window ritual:

REFLECTIONS

Challenges:

One Good Thing:

FASTING

How I felt:

Tough times:

How I did it:

EATING

Opened Window with:

Next, I ate:

Eating pace:

Where I ate:

Closing Window ritual:

REFLECTIONS

Challenges:

One Good Thing:

69   DAY   DATE

FASTED   GOAL   ACHIEVED

WINDOW TIME   OPENED   CLOSED

- 1   2   3   4   5   6   7   8   9   10 +

FASTING

How I felt:

Tough times:

How I did it:

EATING

Opened Window with:

Next, I ate:

Eating pace:

Where I ate:

Closing Window ritual:

REFLECTIONS

Challenges:

One Good Thing:

70   DAY   DATE

FASTED   GOAL   ACHIEVED

WINDOW TIME   OPENED   CLOSED

- 1   2   3   4   5   6   7   8   9   10 +

FASTING

How I felt:

Tough times:

How I did it:

EATING

Opened Window with:

Next, I ate:

Eating pace:

Where I ate:

Closing Window ritual:

REFLECTIONS

Challenges:

One Good Thing:

Week Ten

Reflections

Has fasting highlighted some deeper challenges you may want to address, possibly sugar-addiction, over-eating, stress-eating?

What are some issues you can now see, and what steps might you take to address them?

Have you noticed any effects of autophagy at work? Skin tags, bumps, scars, moles diminishing? Has anyone told you that your skin looks amazing?

Laurie's Corner

"You can't mess this up."

Week Eleven

No Turning Back

- ❯ Notice if your daily fasting practice is awakening new passions
- ❯ Look for areas in your life where you may have given up or stopped doing things you loved in the past.
  - ▸ Friendships
  - ▸ Being in nature
  - ▸ Treats for yourself
  - ▸ Nourishing food
  - ▸ Movement
  - ▸ Handiwork
- ❯ Try on those Goal Jeans and take new measurements

Remember:

1. Keep it simple. There are two parts to every day. The fasting hours and the eating window. Don't make it more complicated than that.
2. Settle in and relax into your groove.
3. Create an environment for support around you.
4. Have at least two other ways to measure your success other than the scale.
5. Keep adding to your WINS list and make sure you have Mantras to stay inspired
6. Know the things you do and say to derail yourself. Don't fall for it.
7. Continue to enjoy the food discovery. Read about the Blue Zones and other healthful ways of living.
8. Go back up to number one, and Repeat.

71 DAY DATE
FASTED GOAL ACHIEVED
WINDOW TIME OPENED CLOSED

- 1 2 3 4 5 6 7 8 9 10 +

FASTING

How I felt:

Tough times:

How I did it:

EATING

Opened Window with:

Next, I ate:

Eating pace:

Where I ate:

Closing Window ritual:

REFLECTIONS

Challenges:

One Good Thing:

72   DAY   DATE
FASTED   GOAL   ACHIEVED
WINDOW TIME   OPENED   CLOSED

- 1 2 3 4 5 6 7 8 9 10 +

FASTING

How I felt:

Tough times:

How I did it:

EATING

Opened Window with:

Next, I ate:

Eating pace:

Where I ate:

Closing Window ritual:

REFLECTIONS

Challenges:

One Good Thing:

---

73   DAY   DATE
FASTED   GOAL   ACHIEVED
WINDOW TIME   OPENED   CLOSED

- 1 2 3 4 5 6 7 8 9 10 +

FASTING

How I felt:

Tough times:

How I did it:

EATING

Opened Window with:

Next, I ate:

Eating pace:

Where I ate:

Closing Window ritual:

REFLECTIONS

Challenges:

One Good Thing:

74   DAY   DATE   **75**   DAY   DATE

FASTED   GOAL   ACHIEVED   **FASTED**   GOAL   ACHIEVED

WINDOW TIME   OPENED   CLOSED   **WINDOW TIME**   OPENED   CLOSED

\- 1   2   3   4   5   6   7   8   9   10 +   - 1   2   3   4   5   6   7   8   9   10 +

FASTING

How I felt:

Tough times:

How I did it:

EATING

Opened Window with:

Next, I ate:

Eating pace:

Where I ate:

Closing Window ritual:

REFLECTIONS

Challenges:

One Good Thing:

76　　　DAY　　　DATE　　　　　**77**　　　DAY　　　DATE
FASTED　　GOAL　　ACHIEVED　　**FASTED**　　GOAL　　ACHIEVED
WINDOW TIME　　OPENED　　CLOSED　　**WINDOW TIME**　　OPENED　　CLOSED

- 1　2　3　4　5　6　7　8　9　10 +　　　　- 1　2　3　4　5　6　7　8　9　10 +

FASTING

How I felt:

Tough times:

How I did it:

EATING

Opened Window with:

Next, I ate:

Eating pace:

Where I ate:

Closing Window ritual:

REFLECTIONS

Challenges:

One Good Thing:

FASTING

How I felt:

Tough times:

How I did it:

EATING

Opened Window with:

Next, I ate:

Eating pace:

Where I ate:

Closing Window ritual:

REFLECTIONS

Challenges:

One Good Thing:

Week Eleven

Reflections

What if eating were a sanctified act? What could that look like? What would you adjust?

Are there aspects of your life that now occur as more holy or sacred?

Is there any "struggle energy" around your fasting? What could you do to release that?

Laurie's Corner

Who has been your favorite teacher, coach, or guide in life? What do you think they would say to you now?

Week Twelve

Next Level

- ❯ Make appointment with health care provider

- ❯ Request access to complete hormone panels to ensure all are in optimal range. If your physician isn't cooperative, you can research "Direct to Consumer Testing" and request your own tests.

- ❯ When you go in for blood work, follow their exact instructions regarding the number of hours fasted you should be. Longer is NOT better. If they say 12 hours, don't fast longer than 12 hours.

- ❯ For the three days before blood work, have longer eating windows. Consider fasting no more than 15-16 hours for those three days.

- ❯ Take a look to see if there is any lingering "diet mindset" in your thoughts or speaking

- ❯ Be sure to flip around the workbook and fill out all the remaining charts, questions, lists, and letters.

78   DAY   DATE

FASTED   GOAL   ACHIEVED

WINDOW TIME   OPENED   CLOSED

- 1 2 3 4 5 6 7 8 9 10 +

FASTING

How I felt:

Tough times:

How I did it:

EATING

Opened Window with:

Next, I ate:

Eating pace:

Where I ate:

Closing Window ritual:

REFLECTIONS

Challenges:

One Good Thing:

79	DAY	DATE	**80**	DAY	DATE
FASTED	GOAL	ACHIEVED	**FASTED**	GOAL	ACHIEVED
WINDOW TIME	OPENED	CLOSED	**WINDOW TIME**	OPENED	CLOSED

- 1 2 3 4 5 6 7 8 9 10 +   - 1 2 3 4 5 6 7 8 9 10 +

FASTING

How I felt:

Tough times:

How I did it:

EATING

Opened Window with:

Next, I ate:

Eating pace:

Where I ate:

Closing Window ritual:

REFLECTIONS

Challenges:

One Good Thing:

FASTING

How I felt:

Tough times:

How I did it:

EATING

Opened Window with:

Next, I ate:

Eating pace:

Where I ate:

Closing Window ritual:

REFLECTIONS

Challenges:

One Good Thing:

81	DAY	DATE	**82**	DAY	DATE
FASTED	GOAL	ACHIEVED	**FASTED**	GOAL	ACHIEVED
WINDOW TIME	OPENED	CLOSED	**WINDOW TIME**	OPENED	CLOSED

- 1 2 3 4 5 6 7 8 9 10 +   - 1 2 3 4 5 6 7 8 9 10 +

FASTING

How I felt:

Tough times:

How I did it:

EATING

Opened Window with:

Next, I ate:

Eating pace:

Where I ate:

Closing Window ritual:

REFLECTIONS

Challenges:

One Good Thing:

FASTING

How I felt:

Tough times:

How I did it:

EATING

Opened Window with:

Next, I ate:

Eating pace:

Where I ate:

Closing Window ritual:

REFLECTIONS

Challenges:

One Good Thing:

83   DAY   DATE

FASTED   GOAL   ACHIEVED

WINDOW TIME   OPENED   CLOSED

- 1 2 3 4 5 6 7 8 9 10 +

FASTING

How I felt:

Tough times:

How I did it:

EATING

Opened Window with:

Next, I ate:

Eating pace:

Where I ate:

Closing Window ritual:

REFLECTIONS

Challenges:

One Good Thing:

---

84   DAY   DATE

FASTED   GOAL   ACHIEVED

WINDOW TIME   OPENED   CLOSED

- 1 2 3 4 5 6 7 8 9 10 +

FASTING

How I felt:

Tough times:

How I did it:

EATING

Opened Window with:

Next, I ate:

Eating pace:

Where I ate:

Closing Window ritual:

REFLECTIONS

Challenges:

One Good Thing:

Week Twelve

Reflections

If you could stand on top of a mountain, or on a balcony overlooking a sea of people, what would you be shouting with joy about? What will you crow about? Bragging is allowed!

What are you most proud of?

(At this point, many people say, "I like black coffee!")

What is the most amazing thing you have accomplished in the last three months?

What don't you ever want to forget?

Laurie's Corner

I am proud of you.

Fast Forever

Troubleshooting

So many pieces of this puzzle have come together beautifully, and you might be chugging along not needing to adjust a thing. Please do not think that you are supposed to change anything. What I wish most is for you is that you are zipping along in life – fasting and eating – and not thinking too much about it.

If this talk of troubleshooting, testing, tweaking, and tinkering is of no interest, then skip this section. Truly. Who needs more stress? Keep it supremely simple. Focus on two things every day:

1. How long will I fast today?

2. What "window worthy" foods am I going to enjoy?

That is it. Two things.

However, if you have intermittent fasted *consistently* for over three months, and are discouraged that you have seen no changes or progress in well over four weeks, it might be time to dig in – bit by bit – and make a few adjustments.

Factors to Consider

- The Clean Fast
  Have you examined thoroughly everything you are consuming during your fasting hours? Are you unknowingly or deliberately consuming anything that is not on the Yes column of the Clean Fast Chart? Go to page 26 and look closely at that list. I have worked with hundreds of people who *swore* they were fasting clean until they noticed Earl Grey Tea is flavored with Bergamot. *Whoopsie!*

- Fasting Timing
  Could you add an hour or two to the length of your fast to take advantage of more fat burning and autophagy? Have you tried one 36:12 per week?

- Food Timing
  Might you be eating to late, and could an earlier eating window work better for your digestion? Is the time of your eating window having you overeat or disrupting your sleep? Insufficient sleep can prevent fat loss.

- Food Quality
  Eating real, whole foods that are not ultra-processed or denatured aids in the healing of the appestat in the brain. Are there foods that you know make you feel better that you could eat more of? Factory-made sugar and treats are not off limits, but is there some aspect of your food choices that you could shift to accelerate your healing and progress?

  Experiment with the balance of macronutrients ("macros") that work well for your body. Not all carbohydrates are created equally! Carbs aren't "bad," and there is a difference between a sweet potato and a bag of cookies. Some people prefer to reduce carbohydrates until they reach their goals, and then gradually reintroduce them.

- Food Quantity
  Are you practicing listening for and respecting the body's satiety cues? Notice when you lean back and *sigh*. That is the body's way of saying, *enough.*

  Practice eating to "80% full," and ask yourself, "am I still hungry?" If the answer is Yes, ask yourself what else you need. Then eat more. If the reply is No, then stop eating. Focus on what your unique body needs day to day, and practice eating to satiety, not beyond.

- Food Allergies & Sensitivities
  Eat what you love, but remember to eat foods that love you back.

  We cannot all eat *everything*. If your body would prefer that you eliminate soy, sugar, alcohol, wheat, dairy, gluten, nuts, meat, or (fill in the blank), then you need to respect that. After all, it is fighting like mad for homeostasis, and you might be creating a lot of extra agony for your body.

  Take away the foods that your body does not want. If that upsets you, you *will* be able to resolve the frustration because feeling better is wonderful!

- Water & Minerals
  Many people go overboard with water, and others do not drink enough. Experiment with switching right over to water after *one* cup of morning tea or coffee. When you are hungry, drink water. Discover the *right* amount for you.

  When insulin is low, the kidneys flush out magnesium and sodium, and drinking excess water can exacerbate this. Therefore, make sure you are adding in enough minerals/electrolytes, especially magnesium.

- Medications
  Are you on any medications that prevent weight loss or cause weight gain?

- Supplements
  Plain magnesium (with no additives) is fine to take while fasting. Try to move most others to the eating window.

- Coffee
  For most people, coffee is an appetite suppressant. But, if you find yourself getting hungry after a cup of coffee, it might be raising your insulin. Keep coffee inside your eating window. Also, for women over 44, too much caffeine raises cortisol and is a strain on the adrenal glands. An abundance of cortisol can store fat, and prevent fat burning. Have one delicious cup of black coffee, and switch to water.

- Diet History
  If you have a history of calorie-restriction and yo-yo dieting, your body will be fixing your broken metabolism before it can address fat loss. This takes time.

- Years Overweight
  Many women have struggled with their weight since childhood. This can lead to a very high level of circulating insulin, and insulin resistance. It takes time to lower the baseline insulin, and it is well worth the time and effort.

- Movement
  You do not need to be a gym rat, or subject yourself to exercise you do not enjoy. That said, how much are you moving your body?

- Deep Dive into Hormones
  Have you had your cortisol, thyroid hormones, estrogen, testosterone, and progesterone checked? Everything in balance?

- Underlying Imbalance or Disease
  Is your body dealing with an autoimmune disease, gut issues, PCOS, etc? Anything that is out of balance will take the body's attention during the fasting hours. These

are your healing hours. Be patient, your body is working for you.

- **Physical Signs**
  Check your waist to hip ratio, or your waist to height ratio. If your belly is disproportionally large, the body is working to reverse inflammation and insulin resistance.

- **Planned Indulgences**
  What do you consider a "special occasion"? How do you define the days when you give yourself some wiggle room to deviate from your plan? As a person who subscribes to the "Delay, Don't Deny" methodology, we aren't interested in deprivation, but, could you tighten up the definition of what "special" is?

- **Your Environment**
  Are your physical surroundings and the people in your life supportive of your intermittent fasting lifestyle? Are you using your calendar to plan, do you have positive alerts in your phone and posted around your desk, car, mirror? Does your family high five you when your window is open?

Looking at the factors above, what speaks to you? Circle or highlight two things that you could you tweak now. Could you:

1. Eat earlier, lengthen your fasting hours, or shorten your eating window.

2. Eliminate or reduce ultra-processed foods. Choose to make fresh, homemade meals. Eating real food might be the only tweak you need. The gut microbiome needs some nutrient diversity.

3. Limit coffee and tea to one cup per day before 10AM.

4. Experiment with Carb Cycling — one day with wholesome carbs on the plate, the next day with mostly fat and protein. Alternate days, carbs on, carbs off.

5. Sleep earlier, and tend to your sleep hygiene practices.

6. Reduce or eliminate alcohol and/or sugar for a period of time. As we move towards menopause, new addictive tendencies (sugar and alcohol) can surface.

7. Plan one or two longer 36:12 fasts per week.

8. Speak with your doctor about your medications.

9. Listen to episode 52 of the Intermittent Fasting Podcast, and request full thyroid panels.

10. Be disciplined in your eating window — practice eating mindfully to satiety, then pausing, and eating again.

11. Look for ways to reduce stress. This is easier said than done, and please don't let the idea stress you out! Meditation, time in nature, early to bed, dancing, etc. Our body can't tap into our fat stores when cortisol is too high.

12. UP your level of engagement in the world of Intermittent Fasting! Read, study, explore, share articles and ideas. You may discover something new about your practice that you can adjust.

Write some ideas here regarding the two things you will tweak.

From _____ to _____
(3-4 weeks from now) I will:

1.

2.

1. You have your 2 Tweaks identified.
2. What do you feel right now?
3. What thoughts are you having about making those adjustments?
4. If you need to reframe or flip those thoughts, write how you will do that now.
5. Jot down your Fasting Mantra, and make sure you are approaching this from a Growth Mindset.
6. Get centered on that Mantra.
7. Fast Forward!

Once those changes are underway, settle in. Resume your stress free fasting pattern and let the body heal and get to work. Make your daily fasting hours be as peaceful as possible, and enjoy your delicious meals.

Only refer back to these lists if you are stuck again. Please do not stress out over an ongoing pressure of troubleshooting and tinkering. Weight loss is a zigzag. When you have some peaceful thoughts about what you might alter, try that. No panic. Be in your fasting flow.

Discouragement

You have heard all of the cliché's regarding quitting, so I will not go there.

But, I want to ask you, what do you have to go back to? Eating small amounts of food all day long, never feeling satisfied, counting & measuring, prepping excess meals and cleaning up, feeling guilty in restaurants, spending unnecessary money, feeling deprived, hungry, fixated and craving, an endless cycle of using food to cope with stress, and being stuck in a hopeless cycle of struggle and anxiety – anticipating being fatter and sicker forever?

There, I said it.

No, I do not think you want to go back to any of that.

I absolutely understand the discouragement and frustration that comes from a plateau, months of seeing "no results." But, remember, this is not a "program," this is exactly how human being's bodies are meant to live. Our bodies *need* to pause from food every day and heal. This is what you need to do, even if you settle back into a 12:12 or 14:10 schedule. You are an intermittent faster.

Right now, take on the mantra that "I know this is good for me," settle into your *stress-free* fasting practice, and fast forward.

You can do it.

It is a good thing we had this little chat. Now, go do something awesome for yourself. Big hugs.

P.S. If the body is not budging whatsoever regarding weight and inflammation, there may be an underlying imbalance or disease that it is addressing. It needs those fasting hours; your fasting is a gift. Please work with your healthcare practitioner to identify the source of the imbalance.

Maintenance

When you get where you are going, you will know when you have arrived. Every intermittent fasting person who has reached *the* place will confirm it is true.

You nail **the** number on the scale, and that is that! Or, you just *know* when you are working in harmony with your body. You may be in a structured, intuitive, informed, insightful, mysterious, flirtatious, awakened flow.

Whether it is the number or a feeling, either way, you can now play around with changing some things. Perhaps, you will experiment with some longer eating windows and different foods. Bottom line, your body will let you know.

For me, I could not imagine living any other way than 20:4 OMAD. Yet, I often have a 14-hour fast on Saturdays so that I can enjoy my favorite hatch chile breakfast burrito at the farmer's market at noon. I don't worry about celebratory weekends or vacations. I have reached my 1,000th day fasting, and I know that however long I fast and however long my eating window is, I will enjoy playing around with it tomorrow.

Now you can start wearing those Goal Jeans, and select a pair of Honesty Pants. That's an article of clothing that has zero stretch, that will always alert you if you need to tighten up your eating window for a week or two.

Through the years you will develop new fasting rituals, timings, and practices that continue to lift you up and support every aspect of your life.

This is a vibrant way to live.

Your Vibrant Future

With intermittent fasting as your foundation, you can count on sustained improvements in your health. You are a person who eats in a pattern of time so that your body can heal every day. Fasting provides a clean canvas for you to have the space and discernment to discover the full spectrum of what your body needs.

- Read through all of the preceding pages and let your accomplishments wash over you.

- Who in your life is fasting? Think of the lives you have changed and will continue to change!

- Imagine the holiday season as an intermittent faster!

- How can this continue to be more and more effortless, and evermore joyful?

Continue to nourish yourself with good nutrition, meditation, spiritual thinking, and time in nature. Move your body, sleep well, enjoy sexual pleasure, foster loving friendships, delve into intellectual pursuits, express yourself creatively... and let's make a deal. How about you let me know how you are doing one year from now?

www.fastforwardwellness.com

Take it From Here: Resources

Of the countless books I devoured over the last 1,000 days, here lie the hallmarks. May they illumine your journey.

Delay, Don't Deny	Gin Stephens, PhD
The Obesity Code	Jason Fung, MD
Feast Without Fear	Gin Stephens, PhD
AC: The Power of Appetite Correction	Bert Herring, MD
Mindset	Carol S. Dweck, PhD
Unmired	Kim Smith
The Biology of Belief	Bruce Lipton, PhD
Atomic Habits	James Clear
Deep Nutrition	Catherine Shanahan, MD
The Miracle of Magnesium	Carolyn Dean, MD, ND
The Yoga of Eating	Charles Eisenstein
Why We Sleep	Matthew Walker, PhD
The Elegance of Simplicity	Sophie McLean
Big Magic	Elizabeth Gilbert
Dare to Lead	Brené Brown, PhD
The Gift	Lewis Hyde

Love Letters to You

The following two pages are dedicated to you. Write a love letter to your future self.

- What do you want to know, remember, envision?
- What have you never told yourself?
- What will bring surprise and delight? What will embolden you?
- Please, take the first page, and write a letter that you will open in three months.
- Fold it over, and tape the corner. Let it work its magic.
- Then, in a few months, when you have wound your way up and down through the first three months of your daily fasting journey, tear it open. Devour it. Contemplate. Reflect. Celebrate.
- 100 days from today, take the second page of blank stationery, date the top, address it to you to read in one year, and write until your heart is full.
- What inspires you, what are you proud of, what awes you about your body, why will you not be stopped by frustration or discouragement, what will you have accomplished in a year's time?

Be generous.

Open this letter in 90 days.

Date:

Dear,

Here I am, at the onset of this journey, writing to let you know...

With Love,

To be opened on:

Open this letter in 12 months:

Date:

Dear,

I have been intermittent fasting for three months. This is what I want for you to know one year from now...

With Love,

To be opened on:

My friend,

Here we are!

I admire you. This really took something, and you stuck with it. Don't you dare, for one second, think you should have done all this "perfectly."

What you have accomplished is out of the ordinary.

Keep going with your enlivening and intentional fasting practice.

You are strong. You bring value to this world in a way that no one else can, and I am happy to share this planet and this life with you. The world is blessed to have your beauty, your voice, your light.

I raise my glass in celebration of your vibrant future. Cheers!

With love,

    Fast forward,

        Laurie

44 to forever

Made in the USA
Columbia, SC
10 March 2020